Auto-Immune Illness:
Playing the Hand
Life Dealt
and
Winning the
JACKPOT!

By Barbara j. Mascio

Published by:

Harmony Publishing
P.O. Box 110331
Cleveland, OH 44111

6/98

Copyright© 1996 by Barbara j. Mascio and Richard Mascio

First printing 1996

Printed in the United States of America

Detroit Avenue Printing, Lakewood, Ohio

ISBN: 0-9653612-4-1, $10.95

Copies of this volume may be ordered by mail or phone directly from the publisher. To order, please include price as noted above plus $3.50 shipping and handling per book. Send to publishers address as noted above. Ohio residents must include 7% sales tax.

DEDICATION

I have shared this story with many people who continually ask, "Please write it down Barb." Based on those requests I began to write this in 1993. I would like to thank all of you who encouraged me to do so.

To thank my Creator almost goes without saying - but I do need to say it. It was learning how to accept, love and find joy in all things, that opened my eyes to the possibility of my living a life full of vibrant health. This came as a gift from God. It was that love that held my family together during the worst of it.

Thank you God.

Had it not been for my husband, Richard, I know I would not have finished the writing of this book. He not only encouraged me, he pestered me. His encouragement and insistence that I keep working on it until completion was just another form of his love and faith in me. Without Richard sharing the entire illness, the subsequent metamorphosis and the re-birth (if you will) of the new me, there would have been nothing to write.

Thank you sweetheart.

Although my son was only visiting on weekends during the worst of the illness, I have to thank him too for his understanding and the amazing ways he was able to behave so unselfishly when so much of the focus was on me and me alone.

Thank you Ross.

ACKNOWLEDGEMENT

Each of us have unique gifts to offer one another. The power of God's Holy Spirit lives within each of us. It is pure light, pure love. We share and we receive it, through one another.

With this in mind, I would like to thank my Earth Angels for always believing in me, for lifting me up, and for saying prayers on my behalf.

(I won't mention what they have done for me. That would be a book in itself!)

Richard, Ross, Pam and Pete Genos, Keith and Betty Simpkins, Pat and Don Mascio, Violet Robbins, John and Charrie Mascio, Pheobe Swain Beetler, Tom Swain, Howard Beetler, Shirley Kelly, Keith E. Simpkins, Jr., Vicky Mascio, Mrs. Villars, Mrs. Cook, Mrs. Zinsmayer, Pastor Ferguson, Cindy and Bobby Matis, Flo Ann France, Christy Shivington, Jim Hogue, Melvin Edmonds, Kathy Burrows, Penny Knight, Jeff Dean, Paul Reynolds, Bridgette Bojaski, Stephanie Bushnell-Morenberg, Sandy Adams, Debi Estes, Charlie & Donna Smith, Karen Barnes, Lauralee Karr, Lorenzo Kane, Michelle Star, Gene and Ann Davis, Francie Dailey, Jackie Cooper, Claudia McWarter, Marsha King, and Dawn Vardrasek, Betty Kleczy.

Thank you for giving of yourself to me and to my family, directly and indirectly. I have no doubt that I have even more Earth Angels that I am unaware of. I apologize if you have not been recognized and excluded by error.

TABLE OF CONTENTS

PART ONE

"The Bowel Ecology"

PART TWO

"Basic Functions"

PART THREE

"The Cellular Level"

PART FOUR

"Water"

PART FIVE

"Oxygen"

PART SIX

"Body Movement"

Conclusion

Product Information

Suggested Reading

INTRODUCTION

This book is my personal journey through Chronic Fatigue Immune Deficiency Syndrome, Irritable Bowel Syndrome, Fibromyalgia (along with a few other ailments). It includes an account of how and why I have chosen the methods described within and how these actions have resulted in my living symptom free!

You, the reader, are welcomed to try what I have proven to myself to work. You may find that all or portions of my methods will work for you.

I am in no way "prescribing" nor giving you advice that would supersede your personal physicians' advice.

If you are reading this, however, I must conclude that you, too, have begun a journey to educate yourself with the hopes of one day benefiting by taking responsibility for your own health. Welcome!

In 1989, at the age of 32, I suddenly awakened to find myself an unwilling participant in a twisted game between life and the darkness. I was angry, depressed, frustrated, terrified and full of doubt.

Your spirit/mind/body are either in the process of dying or they are in the process of healing. My spirit/mind/body, once connected with my Creators' Spirit, began to choose the path of healing. You will see later in this book the definite connections between the spirit/mind/body.

My grandfather was once a coal miner in Pennsylvania. He told stories of the men carrying small birds down into the mines. As a small child, I thought the birds were used for entertainment. I pictured these men working away in dark caves with only the chirping of precious birds to keep them company. I later learned these birds had a much more important purpose. They were used as warnings to the men. A coal miner knew to run for his life if the birds began to show respiratory weakness. The healthy coal miner reacted quickly to save and/or protect himself from environmental poisoning that his body had not yet detected. He knew it would be too late for him if he did wait for the symptoms. Back in those days, when safety equipment was not a necessary commodity those birds saved many lives. My grandfather, who died a grueling death from emphysema, learned, unfortunately, that some environmental poisonings did not manifest themselves as quickly as others.

Those of us who have become ill, our immune systems compromised from any number of factors, whether it is from environmental poisonings, man-made foods, or even antibiotics, might be looked upon as being those small birds. For whatever the reason, we have been given the opportunity to be the "Red Flag of Warning" for the rest of our brothers and sisters, whether human, animal or plant life. By learning how to rebuild our immune system in a fashion to be able to withstand and even co-habitat with new strands of viruses, new and ever-improved chemical poisonings in our environment, we then have the opportunity to teach others how to protect themselves before they feel the symptoms.

I am not an author by trade. I am not a physician. I have learned through trial and error what my body, what any human body, wants and needs. By simply providing the proper raw materials to our spirit/mind/body, we can allow it to follow the path of healing!

I made a promise to God - my Creator - that if I could balance my body I would share all that I had learned with as many as wanted to know. Keeping with that initial promise, I was intent on finding methods that could easily be duplicated. What good is a method if it is too costly to consider? What good is a method if it is so complicated, an ordinary person could not follow the steps?

I believe that what I have done to help myself is simple and easily duplicated. Through reading this book and then by acting on very simple suggestions contained within, you too may begin your way to a healthier tomorrow!

TO YOUR HEALTH - TODAY AND ALWAYS!

> "He that hath a truth and keeps it,
> Keeps what not to him belongs.
> But performs a selfish action,
> And a fellow mortal wrongs."
>
> Andrew Jackson Davis

> *"To become what we are capable of becoming is the only end in life"*
>
> Robert Louis Stevenson

Chapter 1

"THE FLU THAT NEVER WENT AWAY"

November 1989

"What can I do babe?" Richard, my sweet husband, was beside himself with worry. He was sure something more serious than the flu was happening here. He'd never seen me so washed out - so violently ill. "Do you think it may be food poisoning?"

"From what?" I answered weakly as I lie on the couch holding a warm cloth over my eyes. The light, any light, had become so painful I could not stand it. My head was throbbing in pain so severely I just knew something was about to rupture. "I haven't eaten anything you haven't eaten in the past week. If it were food poisoning, wouldn't you have it too?"

"Oh No! Not again!" And with that I was off to the bathroom. I was sick and whatever it was, it was determined to come out of my body from any channel it could find.

"Honey, do you want some Imodium A.D. ™?"

When I look back at that time in our lives, I try to remember all the clues. The clues that could explain when and how and why I became so ill. One of the things I most remember is our immediate response to try anything to arrest the symptoms, to cease the pain. I did not have time to be sick. I had to work. Our family depended on both incomes, as most families do these days.

I remember thinking to myself how "unusual" it was for me to be sick. I kept telling myself, "Man, I'm never sick. I never miss work. What's going on here?"

Truth of the matter was, I never did miss work. But in retrospect, I realize that although I had always managed to hide or suppress the symptoms of an illness, I was never all that healthy. I had just learned to "put it out of my mind." I could work through any "discomfort", any pain. I was almost proud of my stamina and my persistence to work even during my migraines, which I had suffered with for many years.

This time, this flu was different. I did call off work. I had no choice. I could barely move. This flu felt deadly. This flu got my attention.

Eventually, I did go back to work but I never felt "recovered." I went to work and as soon as I got home, I collapsed on the sofa. I didn't even have the strength to eat most evenings. I would sleep until my husband woke me up to go to bed. Some evenings he couldn't wake me enough to get me into bed and he would simply kiss me good night there, fully clothed, and wait until morning to wake me.

My work day had become an undeniable struggle. I had always prided myself at being capable of performing several tasks simultaneously. Suddenly I could no longer do more than one thing at a time. It was as if my concentration was wiped out. If more than one person spoke to me at the same time, which was a normality, all I could hear was static. I felt claustrophobic all the time. I began making dreadful errors in my daily record keeping. I began to lose the ability to do simple math.

I was struggling and fighting back the best way I knew how. I assumed the reason I was losing cognitive thinking was a side effect of my trying to perform with the amount of pain my body was in. I figured all my concentration was focused on trying not to feel the pain and so that was why my mind was not clicking the way it normally did.

I was no longer a pleasant person to work with or for. I had difficulty solving problems when presented by employees. They were losing their faith, their respect, in me as their manager. They were seeing too many mistakes. My employer was experiencing the same conflicts with me as well. I tried to explain, but it all came out sounding like excuses. Especially since I really could not justify any of it except to say, "I'm just not feeling well."

I could not grasp why I wasn't able to snap out of this. I had been on an antibiotic for ten days when I first came down with the flu and since that didn't seem to kick it, the prescription was refilled for another ten days. It just didn't seem to work. I couldn't understand it. Antibiotics had always helped in the past. They were prescribed to me when I had that awful bout with bronchitis a few years back and more recently when I had that case of pleurisy. Medicine always had worked in the past.

I started to think that maybe I was immune to antibiotics from having used them so many times in the past. They had been prescribed for gum infections, yeast infections, ear infections, strep throat and when I was a kid for a lot of different things. Back then if someone in your family was sick with this or that the whole clan was lined up for a dose of penicillin "for our own protection." (Little did I know what the frequent use of antibiotics was doing to my system.)

After a while, three months to be exact, it no longer mattered. I absolutely could not work. The fairest decision for all concerned was that I resign. The truth was, I could not function properly.

I still, at this time, had not come to the full realization that I was very ill. I planned to take a month or so off and rest. Afterwards I would find other employment. Perhaps something less stressful. I had no idea that I would become nearly one hundred per cent house-bound and that the next nine months would be spent in bed. I had no idea at the time that my entire world, as I knew it, was about to die. I was clueless to know that the person who resigned from her job that day would never be seen or heard from again. She, too, was to die.

"All of us are born for a reason, but all of us don't discover why. Success in life has nothing to do with what you gain in life or accomplish for yourself. It's what you do for others."

Danny Thomas

Chapter 2

"THE JOURNEY TOWARD A DIAGNOSIS"

When a person goes to a physician on a regular basis they become that physician's "patient." For any of you who have been through the process of testing to discover what it is that is causing your symptoms, then you know why the word "patient" is used. Patience is mandatory, especially when your very educated well - meaning physician cannot fully explain why you have the symptoms you do.

Quite often one test will indicate that another test must be done. This begins the onslaught of multiple office appointments - testing - specialists - etc. It is extremely distressful on the body, mind, and emotions. With each proposed test, "I'd like to rule out MS", they would say, you have anticipation and fear while at the same time a sense of hope that "something" will show up. Anything was better than not knowing. With each negative test result came confusion, anger, loss of hope, and the feeling you may just be a hypochondriac.

Even when a test result would come back positive, we were left with questions. Irritable Bowel Syndrome was not a condition that would cause memory loss or loss of cognitive thinking. Malabsorption was not an explanation for sound and light sensitivity. Fibromyalgia does not cause a chronic sore throat for two years. All of this left the doctors, myself, and my family quite perplexed.

Each disease, each illness, is described in a text that physicians have at their disposal. In these books are descriptions of all recognized diseases from the National Health Institute, The Center for Disease Control, or some other recognized authority. In order to correctly "give" a patient the name (or the diagnosis) of their disease, the majority of the symptomatology must be proved. This provides the "necessary" label - making way for the "necessary" pharmaceutical therapies.

This makes your physician a bit of a detective who honestly works through trial and error. Any sincere physician will attest to this statement. They are good people with trained observational skills and quite often are able to accomplish their task of diagnosing quite readily.

It is when you present a massive amount of symptoms over a period of time that do not appear to be related that even the best of them will most generally be mystified. This is the puzzlement of Chronic Fatigue Immune Deficiency Syndrome. Even the name of this illness raises controversy amongst the medical society. It has been called many things including the following: Epstein Barr Syndrome, The Yuppie Disease, The M.E. Syndrome, Chronic Fatigue, Chronic Fatigue Syndrome, and many others as well. There are "authorities" in the medical society who continue to dispute this illness altogether and simply believe it does not exist.

The symptomatology of the illness has been confused with Lyme Disease, Fibromyalgia, Clinical Depression, Allergies, Lupus, Irritable Bowel Syndrome, Malabsorption Syndrome and so on.

If you have been the patient of one physician from the beginning of your symptoms and if this physician has been working with you in partnership, that is to say, your doctor listens and believes what you convey to him or her when you describe during each visit how you "feel" then, perhaps, your doctor will be successful in putting together the jig saw puzzle of your many symptoms and determine that you may have CFIDS. At this point, the doctor will have to give you a series of tests in order to eliminate the possibility that your symptoms may be symptomatic of another dreadful illness.

If you have my history then this task will definitely take a great deal of time. I did not obtain a regular family physician until 1989, which made me 32 years old at the time. Prior to 1989 I went to a doctor, any doctor, when I was too sick to forgo a visit, which was usually to an emergency room. A quick check, a prescription, and I was out of there. No regular physicals or checkups. I didn't need that, I was healthy. Why go to a doctor when you're not sick? That was how it was with me. Consequently, no doctor had a record of my health or ill-health.

Making matters worse, I had a great deal of memory loss and loss of cognitive thinking. I had extreme difficulty relaying previous medical history.

I was tempted to simply quit and give up trying. I knew something was wrong, but even the best efforts on my doctors' part proved no certain diagnosis. I was sick of being sick. I was so weary of going to the hospital for tests. The frustration I was feeling is difficult to explain. I thought about allowing whatever was wrong inside my body to simply take over and be done with it. I was not suicidal. I was simply beginning to question, "why bother?"

I would confer with my husband, Richard, who I trusted more than any one person in the entire world. If he had ever indicated in any slight manner, whether it be words or tone of words or even body language, that he suspected that all my symptoms were psychosomatic, then I would have given up trying to help my doctors journey through this maze we were all entangled in. He continued to support me, to enforce with me that there was absolutely no chance of my making myself this ill.

Losing my ability to read and write was horrific. I had been an avid reader all my life and without warning, I no longer was capable. I could read words, but try as I would, I could not make them flow into a meaningful sentence. Thankfully, this is a temporary symptom with CFIDS. It does, however, cycle. It may last for hours, days, weeks or even months. Suddenly it's gone, only to return when you least expect it. Writing, a hobby, a release of mine, would also be impossible for long periods of time. I could not formulate the words let alone transport them through the fingers.

I stopped driving a car when I began to realize I could not remember how I got to where I was going. Prior to that I had given up night driving altogether. I simply could not see.

The pain associated with Fibromyalgia is difficult to relay. It is all encompassing. My skin literally hurt. Turning during sleep would cause such pain I would wake up. It took hours each morning to get moving. Sitting, standing and walking were difficult. It felt like the blood running through my veins was on fire.

The Irritable Bowel Syndrome kept me teetering between diarrhea and constipation. I could no longer tolerate eating raw fruits or vegetables. The resulting colon spasms were insanely and penetratingly horrific.

Assured by Richard to continue with the doctor's plan of action, I kept the doctors appointments and underwent all the testing. Richard was with me through it all.

I have to thank my personal God for this companion of mine. I know many who have this illness who are not so fortunate. He truly was my lifeline. Without him, I may have just allowed myself to perish. Each person afflicted with this or any other life-changing illness deserves a companion like Richard. If you are reading this, and you know of someone who is suffering right now, please, reach out and love them. You may not understand all that is going on and chances are this person is no longer, shall we say, a pleasure to be around, but know this. They need you. Hold them, hug them, listen to their ramblings. You need not say one single word. Just be there for them. God will bless you for your gift.

I also must mention and give thanks for my friend, Flo Anne. Flo Anne and I met because of our connection with CFIDS. We were daily "telephone buddies" for nearly a year before we had a personal visit with one another. To this day, she remains my best friend. And even though she herself was far more sick than I, she was always there for me.

Chapter 3

"THE GOOD NEWS IS, WE KNOW WHAT'S WRONG WITH YOU..."

December 1992

My family physician, armed with tests results from an array of specialists (my file was as thick as the "S" volume of the encyclopedia) suggested I see one more doctor. The latest blood work and throat culture revealed specific antibodies that indicated what she called, "Chronic Fatigue." "Chronic Fatigue?" "You mean the "Yuppie Disease?" I'd heard about this from somewhere. It was what "workaholics" get when they burn themselves out. When they need to sit on the sideline of life. When they get depressed from their lives being so out of balance. " Chronic Fatigue?" How embarrassing. How humiliating. I truly believed that she had reached her limits with me. She could not definitely tell me what was at the root of all the symptoms. She felt a need to appease me by giving my illness a name and now she'd turn my case over to someone who was experienced at treating such clever hypochondriacs. I figured I'd go to him, he would give me a placebo, pat me on the head and send me away.

I laugh now when I remember all these thoughts. Please know I am not the first one, nor will I be the last, to have this conceptualization of CFIDS. A mass portion of the public and a large majority of the medical society has the same notions. Some of your friends and family will too hear this "Chronic Fatigue" label and immediately their thoughts are those of judgment. Their advice to you will be: "Change your lifestyle, slow down, eat more (eat less-some CFIDS people lose weight, most gain), exercise, calm down, sleep more" and so on. The undertone of their advice is full of blame as though, "Well, what do you expect, you've done this to yourself!"

I said little when she was writing out the appointment slip. All words were balled up in my throat. I managed to hold the tears until I was out of the office.

I did keep my appointment the following week, reluctantly, but I did show up.

"Let's see, you have Fibromyalgia, irritable bowel syndrome, migraines, weight loss, low blood pressure, low body temperature, a multitude of allergies. He continued to thumb through, "Uh huh, you have extreme fatigue, light sensitivity, loss of cognitive thinking, short term memory loss. I see. Hmmm, a chronic sore throat, enlarged lymph nodes, noise sensitivity, TMJ, inner ear pain, Malabsorption, hmmm." He skimmed the remainder of the file silently. I sat there, with my sunglasses on, trying to get comfortable.

"I have some questions for you. These are questions I ask of each patient when I'm conducting a screen for CFIDS."

1. "What happens when you exercise?"

- "I can't.

-"Why?"

- "It makes me ill, even walking a flight of stairs can put me back in bed."

2. "Do you feel depressed?"

-"Yes. I can't stand this, I hate this life. I just want to go back to work."

3. "How do you feel in the morning when you wake up?"

-"Exhausted."

-"Do you feel like you slept at all?"

-"No."

4. "Do you wake up during the night?"

-"Only from pain."

-"Explain."

-"Pain, like a migraine, or a colon spasm or just my whole body hurts so much, if I roll over, that pain."

5. "Do you have good days?"

-"Sometimes."

-"What do you do when you have good days?"

-"I try to catch up on everything that's being let go around the house."

-"Then what happens?"

-"I'm usually sick shortly after that. The good days are few and far between."

6. "Do you use drugs or alcohol now, or have you in the past?"

-"No, I don't do drugs, and I don't drink. I did, but that was a very long time ago. Like over ten years or more."

"You may or may not have Chronic Fatigue. I have some specific blood tests I'd like to run for blood counts, antibodies and so on. I would also like to take a urine sample today. No offense, but I'd like to confirm no drug usage today, okay with you?"

"Yes, that's fine."

Then he put his hands on my knees. Looked me straight in the eyes and said, "First, I don't see any indication of this being a case of clinical depression. Clinical depression is treatable with medication and therapy. A clinically depressed person no longer cares about getting well, they make little or no effort at all to change their level of health. All desires to get well are missing because they've given up. You have shown an active interest in getting better, you want to get well. This not the case with true depression."

"However I have no doubt that you are depressed right now. This kind of depression is considered reactive depression. In other words, you would not be depressed if you were not so ill, and ill for this length of time."

It was a validation of sorts and a tremendous load off my shoulders. I suddenly had some faith in this guy. Maybe, just maybe, I had a "real" illness and maybe, just maybe, it was curable.

I left his office, shy of more blood and urine, still weak, still full of pain, but with a tiny spark of hope.

30 days later

The doctor came in and read the blood and urine reports. He read the blood test results out loud. I had no idea what he was saying. The tests did prove, however, that I did have Chronic Fatigue.

"Let's talk about the meds you're taking now. What are they?"

I came prepared for this, as he had asked me during our first visit to remember to bring in every prescription bottle so that he could see it. I began digging into my purse and pulling out the bottles. The various drugs that had been prescribed for various symptoms. The drugs that were suppose to help me. The drugs and the doctors that I had trusted.

I pulled all the medications from my purse. Everything from beta blockers to pain killers to anti-inflammatories and everything in between. After examining each one, no mention was made to discontinue any of them.

"Okay. What I see here clearly indicates Chronic Fatigue Syndrome. Let me tell you what course of action we need to address. First, there is a great deal of research that indicates wonderful results using a small dosage of an anti-depressant. Small amounts taken at night before you go to bed seem to induce a deeper sleep. This of course, allows rest and restoration of the body. It also seems to have the ability to raise the serotonin level which seems to help many patients with their pain threshold. So, I would like to begin you with Zoloft (TM) ."

"Secondly, you will need to learn how to pace yourself. Most of my patients seem to cope well by "doing" activity for 20 minutes and then resting for 20 minutes and so on."

I later learned that in order to be correctly given the diagnosis of Chronic Fatigue Immune Deficiency, it has become widely accepted and approved that first you must meet the CDC list of criteria and be tested to exclude the possibility of it being anything else. The following are the recognized symptoms that would lead a physician to at least begin his or her series of elimination testing in order to correctly give you the diagnosis.

SYMPTOM CRITERIA

Fever

Sore throat

Painful axillary, anterior, or posterior cervical nodes

✓ Unexplained generalized muscle weakness, often worse pre-menstrually

✓ Muscle discomfort, myalgia or fibromyalgia trigger points

Prolonged (24 hours or greater) generalized fatigue after levels of exercise that would have been easily tolerated in the patients' pre-morbid state

New or different generalized headaches

Migratory arthralgia without joint swelling or redness

Neuropsychologic complaints (photophobia, transient visual scotomatat, forgetfulness, excessive irritability, confusions, "brain fog", difficulty thinking, inability to concentrate, depression)

Sleep disturbance (hypersomnia or insomnia)

Description of the main symptom complex as initially developed over a few hours to a few days

Frequent findings include:

Depression (occurring since the onset of illness)

Recent onset of food and/or environmental allergies

New onset of digestive disturbances

Increased sensitivity to temperature extremes

Recent onset of menstrual disturbance

My visit with the doctor continued.

"Do you have any questions?"

"How did I get this?"

"There are many theories at this time, but the truth is, no one really knows for sure."

"How do we cure it?"

"Chronic Fatigue is not a curable illness. You have a good chance of it going into remission however. In fact, studies have shown that after 5 or 6 years, a large portion of CFIDS patients seem to recover to about 65% of their original energy levels."

"Are you sure I don't have AIDS?"

"Have you been at risk?"

"I have been monogamous with my husband for 7 years, since we've been together. Prior to that, who knows what I may have been exposed to?" (I was remembering some of my past, a lousy first marriage, a rape, dating in the '70s when "Love the one you're with" was the motto)

"Have you ever shared a needle?"

"No. I've never used a drug with needles."

"Testing you for HIV would be a good idea. Just to rule it out and to give you some peace. However, I do have to ask you to sign a consent form. Although the results of your test may never need to become public, the fact that you're being tested at all, puts up a Red Flag to the insurance companies as it says you may be at risk. Now legally, they cannot cancel your coverage, but you never know."

He went on to try to pursued me to have the test done anonymously at a clinic, but I was too tired and I just wanted to get the test over with. I kept thinking, as he was talking, how if I had not appeared to be this nice white middle class lady living in a western suburb, how the question for possible HIV would most likely have been made by him, hell, by any one of the doctors I had seen over the past years.

Ever been tested for HIV? The blood technician reads his paper, what you're being tested for and his whole demeanor changes. It's an empty silence filled with curiosity, fear and disgust. You feel compelled to fill the silence with chit chat but you can't think of a thing to say. You watch his eyes. Searching for some compassion. Even for a sign of professional impartiality. What you see is concentration on the needle. No room for a slip here. Gloves, masks, protect him from you. Nothing protects you from him. The test takes seconds, you'll swear you're alone with him for hours. You pray you'll never see this technician again. God forbid he knows someone you know.

Testing for HIV is traumatic. Waiting for the results are, well, words cannot describe it. Please. Love, like you've never loved, any one you meet who is HIV positive. Love those with AIDS. Their journey is unthinkable . They receive the same scorn as those afflicted with leprosy back in the Old Testament. Think of how we look at that affliction now and how we shake our heads at the unlovable uncaring people who mistreated them. How we are amazed at their stupidity in their reaction to leprosy. I believe, years from now, people in the future will have the same revelation of this thing called, AIDS.

Receiving the news that I was negative was a relief, yet there was a feeling that HIV negative test results would not be a certainty of not having AIDS. The symptomatology of AIDS, so publicly reported on in recent years, were undeniably a mirror image of many of the symptoms found in CFID's. AIDS means, Acquired Immune Deficiency Syndrome. CFIDS means, Chronic Fatigue Immune Deficiency Syndrome. Hmmmmm.??? Needless to say, I did not have the same celebratory reaction as my doctor.

The testing was complete. No cure. Treatment included pharmaceutical therapy and learning how to pace myself. I would be expected to continue to have my condition monitored. I should begin looking forward to remission one day with the C.F.I.D.S. but I should expect only a 65% return of who I was and even that would have to wait for the remission year, if, that is, I was one of the lucky ones to reach remission.

Receiving a death sentence would at that time, have been easier to digest. I wanted this pain to end. I could not see to the end of it and my doctor wasn't promising an end.

I was pissed.

Not satisfied with the information provided to me by the doctor (s) I began to search for written material about this illness. I highly recommend the following books on this illness as it will show you what you are up against. It is always prudent to be aware of your adversary.

"What Really Killed Gilda Radner?" written by Neenyah Ostrom
"The Canary and Chronic Fatigue Syndrome" written by Dr. Majid Ali
"50 Things You Should Know About The Chronic Fatigue Syndrome Epidemic" written by Neenyah Ostrom
"Osler's Web" written by Hillary Johnson

"We must never forget that we may also find meaning in life even when confronted with a hopeless situation, when facing a fate that cannot be changed."

Viktor E. Frankl

Chapter 4

SURVIVING A METAMORPHOSIS

I was raised to be a fighter. The words, "I can't" were not part of my vocabulary. I had always prided myself with that. I was also a "worker." I was an employers dream ... I was dedicated, a team player and loved challenges.

I had also been raised to believe, "Idle hands are the Devil's play" and "He's not worth his salt" and "A job worth doing is worth doing right." (and so on)

I had developed no hobbies. I spent no time cultivating friendships. My life, my definition of who I was, was all wrapped up in the work place. This is where I navigated. I was good at it and received all my strokes there. The very validation that I "counted" for something was focused in the workplace.

Relationships

My sisters and I had created a drama with one another years ago as children. They looked at me as the "strong" one, the one who never needed anything. They came to me with their problems, emotional and financial, all their lives and I was always their rescuer. I was never a "sister." I was more to the extreme of a doting mother. The kind of mother who was constantly trying to fix your problems in a way that didn't allow you the opportunity to handle your own problems in your own way. I always knew the "best" way and although they came to resent this character in me, they, for many years, helped to create it. In all our lives, not one of them were ever available to be the "giver" in my life. This illness did not prompt them to change their role with me. This hurt me in the beginning. I came to understand, much later, that I had unrealistic expectations of them and of our relationship.

Once, after the first few months of being house-bound, I actually called one of my sisters who lived one block away. I said to her, "You know, I have always been there for you no matter what and here I am in real need. Why can't you come over and at least help me clean the house or do up a load of dishes?"

Her reply, "No one can stand to be around you when you're sick Barb, you are just too bitchy."

The very first baby steps towards acceptance

Yes. Bitchy covered it. I was. I was so angry. My entire life as I knew it no longer existed and the doctors were telling me not to expect it to return. They were telling me, at age 33, to give up, accept it and file for disability.

I was sorry that I wasn't terminal. I know this sounds very self-ish but this is honestly what was going through my mind. I share this personal part of my journey not to gain sympathy but because I don't believe I am the only one who went through this part of the mourning process. I have a feeling that sharing some of my "ugli-ness" will be helpful to those who are also feeling like this and are ashamed of it. My message to you, don't be ashamed. If you are experiencing an emotion, that emotion is real. Recognize it. Give yourself the permission to feel it. You'll learn how to let it go when it's time for you to let it go.

These were some of my inner most thoughts ...

I was actually "wishing" that the final diagnosis would be one of a terminal disease. Not that I wished to die, per se. I just could not imagine feeling like this or living this way forever. I also "wished" that my illness could be one of some respectability, like a cancer or lupus or something with a "label" so that when people heard it they would not only recognize it, they would be, if not sympathetic, at least they would be empathetic. If I had cancer, my family would have easily been able to "excuse" my bitchiness. They would have attributed that to the cancer and they would not have left me so alone. They would have been there with me.

Not only did I find myself "house-bound", a kinder more gentler way of saying that I had become a shut-in, I felt so abandoned.

This is not to say that all family and friends disappeared from our lives by their choice. Rich and I kept many of the details of the illness from those we felt a need to protect. We didn't want to worry them. Not wanting people to see me in this state, I also went out of my way to discourage visits.

I developed a kinship with a family the local news had been reporting of, whose college daughter suddenly came up missing, during this time in my life. There were no clues. No ideas, whatso-ever, to where she was. And worse yet, who may have abducted her. Or why, or even if she was still alive. I watched the eyes and the faces of the family and friends of this beautiful, talented young woman, as they were being interviewed. Tears of desperation with quivering voices filled equally of doom and of hope.

The reports hit the news, off and on, for nearly a year. It eventually was no longer the lead-in story, it became a little bleep of a few seconds, somewhere between the weather and the high school sport scores. She's still missing.

Please know, that this following analogy is not meant to trivialize their pain or on the other hand to somehow elevate my pain. But what they were going through, this weird type of sadness and mourning, is what I was feeling for my life. It's what every single person I have talked to feels like, who would rather be working and instead find themselves house-bound for an indefinite period of time. Let me try to explain ...

Death is permanent. (At least on our side of the gates) It's sad, but we know what to do about it. We might feel some initial denial, anger, grief and even rage. But eventually, we learn how to accept the loss and move on. But when something as horrible as an abduction happens, what do you do? Giving up hope that this person will be found is down right sacrilegious. How could a parent do that? And yet, ask yourself, "How many months, how many years need to pass before the hope dies?" When do you finally have to believe that this person is not coming back? I don't think you can do it that way. Yet, you have to come to terms with it enough to where you are able to "live" your life. Find peace and happiness, somehow, despite the hard facts that part of you, part of your very being, your child, is "gone." Not dead, not where you know where the tomb stone is. Where the body is. Not anything quite as real as that. Just ... gone. You also know, because your hope as a parent will never let you believe this child won't someday be found, that when that day happens, the child you knew, the child you last hugged, that child, will never, ever, ever come home. When your child is found, she may be dead. You're somewhat prepared for that. We all know, how we do that one. The fears that permeate your every breath though, is wondering if the child will return, completely different, damaged, scared from the inside out from her ordeal.

And yet, you have to keep "hope" alive. Anything short of that would mean your faith had died. Once you allow you "faith" to die, you know you'll be totally alone. A loneliness already cloaks your home from the isolation that must occur in a situation like this, from all relatives, neighbors and friends. Oh, I'm sure they are right there with all their well-meaning words, hugs and casseroles in the beginning. But as time passes they run out of things to say. They most likely become impatient with you. They move on, you are stuck with no place to move on to. That begins to make them uncomfortable around you. So they stop calling. They stop inviting you places. They ease their conflict by telling themselves, "It's best we don't upset them. It's best we just stay away right now."

And so it is with those of us with chronic illnesses, those of you who were forced into early retirement, and I would venture to say, the larger portion of the elderly population. All of us who loved to work and no longer are able or allowed to.

You see, as we come to terms with our new life, the one we are now "forced" to live - not the life we had aspired to live, we mourn who we once were. We hold on to hope as fiercely as a warrior holds to their shield that someday, somehow, the person we used to be, will come back. Back to our family, to our friends, to our co-workers; to all the people in our lives dependent on us financially, emotionally and physically. We don't want this type of existence, we want our lives back, just the way it was. And we suffer the pain of isolation when friends no longer know what to say. When relatives get impatient with us, waiting for us to "snap" out of it. When we ourselves push well-meaning people away with our anger at ourselves.

On the surface, it may seem that our mourning is ego-driven, that we're suffering over the loss of a more vital body, a clearer-thinking mind, our jobs. It is not that simple. We have lost the very definition of who we are. The very essence of our lives has, in all reality, disappeared. We can live with the physical limitations left to us, but we continue to yearn for "who" we once were. Just as I'm certain this family would welcome home their daughter, in any mental and physical condition, they would indeed continue to mourn over the loss of her once innocent self, her essence of "who" she was prior to the abduction.

So, I wasn't "terminal." That meant I would live but live a different life. I tried to assure myself that this might be a tremendous opportunity. I rarely believed myself.

I am fortunate in that my husband, Richard, is out of pure love and friendship, continuously open to listening to my thoughts, my anger, my confusion. And he too continues to contemplate and offers an insight that only a very wise old soul would possess. Sadly, many marriages dissolve, with one spouse suffering with their own personal dragons and the other spouse unable to relate and unwilling to remain part of it. I was blessed with my mate.

Prior to the illness, Rich and I shared each others' day, the work day, with one another with genuine interest. He knew what was going on in "my" world and I his. After the news that I would not get better and that I would not be able to return to work, in addition to being self absorbed in trying to adjust, I totally lost interest in Richard's world. I didn't want to know what was going on with him outside of our home. I wasn't part of that world and I was, I think, jealous. I couldn't bear to hear of his "productivity", I could not stand to hear of his goals and the working of those goals.

He would come home and find me angry. For months on end. He'd come in, bend down, kiss me, and say, "How was your day, babe?" At first I would try to answer as pleasantly as possible for me. But one day I just let him have it. I said, "How the @#%@! do you think it was? It was the same as yesterday. I laid here all day and got up to go to the bathroom. That's it. The house is a wreck and I can't do it!" and then I continued to vent for some time, rambling on and basically exploding all over this wonderful - loving - concerned - worried man.

Very wisely, he sat beside me, held my hand, and let me go. He said nothing. When I was finished, he simply said, "I love you Barb. Do you know how very important you are to me?"

He never asked me how my day was after that. He understood. I had become an unwilling spectator and I did not want to live his life as a way of living my life. I wanted a life of my own.

A few months from this point I began to believe the doctors might be right. This just might be the way my life was going to be. I love Richard more than words can say and I just could not picture allowing this wonderful man to "care" for me like this for the rest of our lives. I began a logical campaign to convince him to divorce me. At first I was very kind about it. I explained that it would be the best thing for all of us. I would not feel guilty about him "having" to take care of me and he would be free to live a life. A life free of me - the burden. He reacted to this as lightly as possible. Choosing to play it like I was kidding. So, I became more insistent. Bitchy doesn't even begin to cover it. But he would not hear of it.

I could not comprehend why he would not take me up on this. I loved him and I didn't want his life to be this way. I knew he loved me but he could still love me and not be forced to stay in this marriage.

This part is really personal, but those with chronic illnesses will relate. Sex was not part of our lives. I don't mean it was cut down in frequency, I mean it did not exist. I was in so much pain all the time that it was out of the question. I also went through a fearful period of wondering whether or not Rich could actually contract, if not the whole illness, one of the viruses that I was carrying.

Our sex life had always been special to both of us. We loved making love to one another. Our relationship was not centered on sex, thank God. But it was a very enjoyable part of our lives.

I continued to relinquish ...

So, there I lay, all day, totally alone. I couldn't read. I didn't have the "comprehension" to even follow a silly TV show. No one was visiting. No one was calling. Rich worked his normal 9 to 10 hours a day. And I lay there with only my mind to keep me company and at that point, my mind was my own worse enemy.

I was beginning a journey, a metamorphosis. One without promotions, one without deadlines. One without the paycheck. I found it, quite literally, terrifying. How would I measure myself without the recognition of a promotion or a pay raise? What inner glory could I possibly feel with no deadlines to accomplish, no bottom line to effect? What would I possibly have to talk about at the end of the day? How would I ever feel whole?

Without my best friend, without Richard, I do not know how I would ever had unraveled the questions and the answers. (I now know that God was at work in my life and worked through Richard but I didn't feel too close to God at that time. I was actually quite angry at God) But without Richard to talk to, to vent, to converse with on any level I was at at the moment, I do not know how I would have survived.

It was during one of our talks when I was going on and on about my struggle to re-define myself now that Rich offered the following insights:

"From the time you are a very small child, adults start asking the question, "What are you going to BE when you grow up?" And children answer with, "A fireman, a policeman, a doctor, a teacher" etc. If you, as a child would answer, "I'm going to be a kind and giving person who loves my family and my friends. I'm going to be a great son or daughter or a dedicated husband or wife. I'm going to work at being spiritually enlightened and use my artistic talents to make this a better world." You would have received a "look" and the question would have been repeated, like you must have misunderstood, until you answered with the "right" answer, the expected answer, a correct definition of who you were to BE.

But it doesn't end there. We continue to grade ourselves by the successes within our occupation. Recognition in the form of promotions, pay raises, being vested within the administration, hugs from the students, praises from the parents.

As an adult, in your occupation (a childhood dream come true or just where you ended up due to circumstances) when you introduce yourself to someone new and they ask, "What do you do?" They don't want to hear, "I play with my kids, I spend quality time with my wife." They want hear - what do you do to make money.

It reasons then, that we as a people create a world with the obnoxious expectations of "what we do" is "who we are." It is how we "measure" up, to ourselves and to others. Certainly we leave the imprint of who we are in everything we do, with every person we meet, with every occupation, with every day we live. But is it fair to our children, to ourselves, to only measure who we are by what we do?

Being ill does not change who you are. It simply changes what you do for a living."

This living room psychology suddenly caused a light to go off in my mind. I had been struggling with how to define myself, how to measure myself, how to accomplish anything my family would find pride in. The constant nagging worry of "who am I now?" You know what? "Who" I am, had not changed just because "what" I do had been altered.

I further realized that I'd been wasting a lot of time and energy mourning over the loss of "What I did for a living." Who I am now is who I have always been. My expectations and my perception of the "who" had always been focused and measured by my career. That no longer exists. Therefore, I now am faced with the challenge of personifying who I am through new avenues and undiscovered routes, ones not defined by "occupational titles."

Simple? Yes, it really is. An easy task? I should say not! We're actually talking about re-programming thought processes ingrained within me since I can first remember.

I was raised in a middle class blue collar family with multi-generational ties to "an honest day's work for an honest day's pay." I cannot remember anyone in my family ever being on welfare or unemployment or on disability. Work is everything in my family. Work outside of the home and work inside the home. Time was spent on teaching good work values, time was spent in school to learn how to get a better job, time was spent at work to learn how to better yourself. Conversations in the home were work-related.

I learned the importance of being on time, "putting your best foot forward", to never complain unless you had a solution, to have respect for those holding positions below and above you, to ask questions and so on and so on. Great life lessons, but they were all tied into the work world.

I can't ever remember an adult in my life just taking the time to learn to play an instrument - just for the fun of it. Or to listen to music - just for the sheer pleasure of the music and not to be used as background sound while they attended to a chore. Or to allow themselves the pleasure of just ... being. Allowing themselves to read for the entertainment value as opposed to the need to not "waste time" and to only read books that added to their education. Or even to just .. play. Play with no reason, just play.

As a child I quickly learned that successful adults were busy adults. Sitting still, day-dreaming, playing with no educational value, was somehow, wrong. I realize now, that developing that side of me means removing the immediate sense of guilt I feel when I am doing, for all apparent perceptions, nothing. Or in other words, when what it is I am doing will ultimately produce nothing tangible. Nothing materialistic, nothing you can touch or take to the bank or hang on the wall, or brag about at the next family gathering.

There's more to me, there's more to you, there's more to all of us, than the definition we have placed on "who" we are based on how we have titled or defined our occupations. Your occupational title does not describe WHO you are.

I AM

I am
not defined by
my occupation
address
clothes
income
education
music

I am
more defined by
my intangible
esoteric
immaterial
assets

Honesty
loyalty
humor
love

It is the way in which I do things that defines me,
not the things that I do.
The way movies choke me up

The joy I feel when you laugh

The warmth I feel when we're close

The desire I have to care for you

It is these and more that define me

If another had the same material possessions and job

We would still be two distinctly different people

I am I

Richard 11/95

Creative discovery began ...

And so the transformation was beginning for me. The letting go of the workplace was somehow more difficult than coming to terms with the illness. I came to a place where I knew I was being presented with an awesome opportunity. One that would afford me the luxury of being able to completely redesign my life. I was not the old Barb. I was not yet the new Barb. I was in the middle of being able to create the new Barb. How frightening. How thrilling.

As I cycled through this path my health remained basically on the same level. I would have "good" days, though far and few between. My cognitive thinking which was paramount to whether or not I could read or write, would cycle. Some days I had it, some days I didn't.

When I did have cognitive thinking I learned to take advantage of it and began experimenting with activities that I might find as an avenue to express myself, thereby define the new Barb.

I would write. A release and therapy for myself. A unique way to express oneself. I learned to pick up colored pencils, chalks, paints and just create. I learned how to crochet afghans.

Had I never become ill, I would never had known these were things I can do! Things I honestly enjoy doing. I didn't know this creative being was in there.

I learned something very valuable. A truth I would like to share with you. I have come to believe that encouraging the creative being in you is absolutely essential to finding who you are. It is a step in healing that, for me at least, could not be overlooked. Being free to create or in other words, to express your inner most self, is the fulcrum in the balancing of ones health.

I believe the words in the Bible where it says our Creator created us in their image. Being a creation of a creator implies (strongly) that we also must be creators. I believe beyond the "pro-creation" status. We are to express with creativity who we are. You can do this with crafts, hobbies, dance, song. You can do this with re-arranging or re-decorating your home. Find a way to discover your creativity. Play, create, laugh. Laughter can be a creative way to express oneself. Not little smily giggles - but real belly laughter. Laughter that can bring tears.

How can creativity be expressed with laughter? With your imagination. With learning to see life with a comic twist instead of a tragic twist.

Have you forgotten how to laugh? (Smirking does not count!) I know. I've been there too. Laughing at yourself as you move between the bed and the toilet is not an easy task. Some of you, like me, might have to go out of your way to create laughter.

Enlist all who are with you in this illness and explain your need to help finding things to laugh at. As you are on a search for laughable stimuli ask them to also be on the look. Start clipping funny cartoons, humorous cards, bumper stickers, funny buttons and so on. Look for comedy videos, ones you can buy and have the ability to slip into the VCR at times when you can't get to a video store. Collect comedy audio tapes.

As you collect these things, use them. Tape up different humorous sayings or pictures all over your house. Surround yourself with laughter triggers.

Why is creativity so necessary? Why is laughter so necessary? Because these "brain" activities HEAL you. I have read many theories focusing on the healing phenomenon on the cellular level with laughter. I read of actual laboratory experiments proving what has been known since the Old Testament times. In one such experiment, they took a group of people and stimulated them to laugh so hard tears were made. They collected these tears and ran tests on them. They took the same group and stimulated them to the point of sadness until tears came. They collected these tears and also ran tests on them.

The tears from laughter were full of chemicals that were found to be immune enhancers! The tears from sadness were, on the other hand, full of chemicals that were found to break the immune system down. This is scientific fact. Your sadness is hurting you. And I know you don't feel like laughing when you're sad. That's why I recommend you surround yourself with objects and toys and stimuli and creativity that will actually trigger laughter. You need to laugh.

My writing became a channel of sorts. I would create a character or circumstance that would represent me and my question, yet it wouldn't be me. I could look at that person I made up and help them ask questions and from no where (and from everywhere) answers would come to their (my) questions. It was great therapy for me.

The beginnings of a joyful existence ...

I learned through my writing how to accept and yet not totally give in to this illness. Answers would suddenly appear on paper from my pen. I believe this was a blessing, a gift. I learned to relax and listen to truths and to simply allow.

I believe there are no original thoughts. Your thoughts may seem unique to you, but sooner or later, you will discover someone or several who have had the same basic thought.

Some describe this phenomenon of "hearing" answers the process of connecting into the collective consciousness. Others say it is the result of your spirit directly connecting with Creators' Spirit.

I was not aware of "how" this was happening. I didn't plan, or learn or study "how" to do it. It just happened. I am so grateful.

I learned it was okay to have physical limitations. I discovered that it doesn't matter how wide my circle of life was. What mattered was what I chose to fill my little circle with. In other words, I slowly stopped mourning the old Barb.

I learned to stop asking "Why?" and learned to say, "Why not?" I learned to stop pondering or more to the point, obsessing, over what the purpose of my life was. Oh, we all go through that. Why am I here? What's my purpose?

I highly recommend reading "Man's Search for Meaning" written by Dr. Vicktor Frankl. He suggests rather than pursuing the meaning of life in that way, simply turn the question around. Instead of asking "What is my purpose?" ask, "What is life asking of me?"

I took that piece of advice and used it. I saw how totally egotistical I was being. What if my purpose in this life was meant to effect someone else's life and it was that simple. In other words, my purpose for being here may have been as uncomplicated as a chance meeting with a stranger on a bus some 10 years ago who's life was changed by our conversation.

I used his advice and actually changed it a bit. I began asking, "What is life asking of me - TODAY?" I had to do that. I could not see past the todays without experiencing anxiety. And I began to answer the question each day. An example, today life may have asked me to do something as simple as cuddle my son or hug my husband. My "mission" for the day, what life was asking of me, may have been so basic as to do the laundry or bake banana nut bread.

The key in all of this is to do what life is asking of you with a "joyful heart!" When life asks of you to do, let's say the laundry, wash, dry and fold with a happy and thankful heart. If you do the laundry resentfully wishing that you could be out in the corporate world or out saving the world you'll miss the whole thing. "Be" where you are in that moment and live it as though it is the last moment of your life.

You know the poster that says, "Today is the first day of the rest of your life!" Change that to say, "Today is the last day of the rest of your life." Watch and see your priorities change. Watch and see your attitude towards life itself change. Watch and see the patience you'll have with your tongue. Who wants to leave their last impression with people as being a grumpy old you know what.

It somehow took a tremendous load off of my mind to not have to continually search for "my" purpose. I know I have one, I don't know what it is. But it simply doesn't matter. As long as I ful-fill the request of what life is asking of me today and each day and fulfill those requests with a sense of purpose, love and acceptance then I am living a meaningful life. A strange thing will start to occur to you, if you decide to try this. A few months will pass and you will suddenly become aware of a sense of "purpose" a sense of "fulfillment." Why? Because after many days of giving to life what it has asked of you, those days add up and you look back at it with the eyes of retrospect and you see, quite magically, that you are fulfilling your purpose. You know you are, even if, like myself, you cannot yet "define" what it is. You just know. Please try this, it brings such peace and you can do this, regardless of your current health status. Why do I know that? Because your life will not ask of you something you cannot give or do at your present moment.

SEARCHING FOR THE PURPOSE
by Barbara Mascio

God planted a seed in a bed of sand
to see what it would do,
No sun, no soil, no nourishment,
It sprouted ... and it grew.

The roots were short and very weak,
Yet the stalk was oh so strong,
Void of buds and missing leaves
Different ... but not wrong.

The seasons entered in and out,
The plant refused to die,
So full of life, so full of hope
Forever searching ... asking why?

Growing this way, stretching that,
Thick with dew it cried,
It wanted answers for this life,
The beauty was ... it tried.

Then the mind monsters came to further the healing...

Being alone was something I had never done correctly in my entire life. I am the oldest of three sisters and part of a large step and half brother and sister family. From there, I joined the Army. Then I got married and had a child. During the divorce that ensued with my first husband, I was thrown into "aloneness", especially when he took my son from me during an ugly custody battle, but I ran from that. I am ashamed to admit, that I ran right smack down the neck of a vodka bottle. I could not be alone. I was not divorced for a full two years before re-marrying. Still, not having custody of my son, the silence that replaces the chatter of your child, the emptiness facing you on the front of the refrigerator because he's not there to draw for you today, was a haunting aloneness for me. I filled the aloneness that time, not with drink, but with work and activity. I had never faced being alone and allowed myself to live it.

This illness forced that on me. I was alone. I could not run from it. I was too smart now to drink. I didn't have the physical strength to "busy" myself with activity. I had to, for the first time in my entire life, listen to my thoughts.

This was hell. I mean that. Hell. All the years of pain, of guilt, of hate, of anger, all neatly suppressed and "forgotten" about, finally had the opportunity to not only get my attention, but to dominate it. I could not shut it off. A cleansing of my mind, of my spirit was going to happen whether I wanted it to or not.

It was during these times that I chose to let it come. I decided it was time to deal with this stuff. I was still secretly harboring the fear that I may indeed be dying and the doctors may have just missed a tumor meshed in the brain somewhere. Who wanted to die with unfinished business? Who wanted to die without forgiveness or without forgiving those who hurt me?

I've never been certain about the theory of reincarnation, but I do believe in a life after this one. Why start that life out with the deficit of this one? So, I buckled down and began to sort it all out.

I discovered I held tremendous guilt over things I did or didn't do or things I said or didn't say during the years of my childhood. Things that I could not be or should not be held responsible for. An example: I felt overwhelming guilt over not taking better care of my sisters. I am one year older than one of them, two years older than the other and five years older than the last one. I was harboring guilt over inadequacy on my part with events in our lives that occurred when I was six. So, this six- year- old held the guilt because she failed the five- year-old? How utterly silly. I had to look at that six-year-old, not as being me, but as the nurturing mother of me and say, "Barbie, you were six. Honey. Let it go sweetheart. You had no control over the situation. Sweetie, you were a mere child. There was nothing you could have done. Your crime is that you were too hard on yourself. Would you expect your son, at age six, to feel that responsible for let's say, his cousins? Of course not. Now don't you see how silly you are being with yourself?"

Don't laugh. I did have to play these dramas out in my mind as different characters. Sometimes I was a nurturing mom, sometimes I was this uninvolved detective interested in just the facts. Nothing else. This detective was able to shed light on many misconceptions I held that kept me poisoned with self-blame and guilt. Man. Did I have a lot of guilt to purge.

Loosing custody of my son. Wow. What a guilt trip that was for me. The detective was able to show me how that all happened. And that given the same set of circumstances it would happen again. Why? Because I did not have the life skills back then that I have today. I did my best with what I had to work with. I couldn't have done anything different.

And I continued with my healing. I "forgave" myself for being human and let it go. But the stuff I did, whether intentional or not, that hurt people and hurt myself that I rightly had guilt feelings over, I had to give to my Creator. I had to ask my Creator for forgiveness and ask for the guidance in how to forgive myself. I also had to ask the forgiveness of those I hurt and try to make some kind of amends to them. If making amends wasn't appropriate (people I had long lost touch with) then I looked for some other person in my life that I could give something of myself to.

Now. How to deal with all the anger and hurt feelings I was harboring with people who had hurt me? This was an absolute must. I had to let these things go. I understood how the only person I was hurting was me. I just didn't know how to let it go and I wasn't sure why I should.

It's a difficult thing, letting someone "off the hook" when they have never recognized what they did to you in the first place. When you know you will never hear an apology from them. Staying angry, remaining hurt, was my way of never letting them off the hook. It helped me to justify some of my "weirdness" because I could always point to an abuse of some sort and say "I wouldn't be this way if that wouldn't have happened to me."

And of course I was right. I was the sum total of all of my experiences and being a "survivor" of abuses such as I had gone through gave me certain labels that elicit a certain degree of empathy from those around you who know of your background. I had come to believe (somehow) that letting them off the hook without hearing an apology was almost like saying it didn't really happen or it didn't really matter.

But I'm here to tell you, holding onto hate, anger, fear and all the other personality quirks that these and other negative emotions fuel, will damage you. Not only the emotional and spiritual planes, but also the physical, bringing actual damage to your cells, to your immune system.

Your cells hold memory, not just of DNA and other biological matter, but emotional memory. When you "feel" a memory, a happy one or a sad one, your body's memory (in a way) rewinds itself to the moment you initially had the experience that created the memory. Your body reacts by producing the same kinds of chemicals it did the first time.

What this said to me was this. By choosing to keep harmful memories alive, I was choosing to allow my body to continue to dump toxic harmful chemicals into myself that aided in breaking down my immune system.

I also came to this realization on another level. Originally, when the bad thing (s) happened, I was the victim. By continuously choosing to connect myself mentally with the experience, I was continuously allowing myself to keep the role of "victim." I had to realize that I was not their victim any more, how could I be, we didn't live in the same house, we didn't even see one another any more. I was giving my oppressors power over me for years without them having to make one move.

I realized another truth. I was addicted to anger. To guilt. To anxiety. To fear. Truly addicted. These addictions were the very culprits who steered me towards self-destructive behavior and self-abusing mental thoughts.

I further realized that I was the only person in this whole world who could be responsible for my thoughts. I created them and gave them life. I could un-create them and exchange their lives for other non-destructive thinking, if I chose to.

So. What to do about the forgiveness? In order to make myself healthier I needed to forgive (and hopefully - forget). It's pretty hard to go up to someone and tell them you forgive them when they haven't ever acknowledged what they did and obviously haven't asked for forgiveness. Doing it that way, could actually create a confrontation, a confrontation that would have proven to be non-productive for either of us.

This is how I did it. I would sit (or lay) and use my imagination. I would first picture myself sitting under a big tree in the middle of this beautiful safe meadow. Once I felt quite comfortable and safe and most importantly, in control of the situation, I would "bring" the person into the scene who I wanted to forgive. I would "bring" them in at quite a distance from where I sat. I would creatively move them closer to where I was. Sometimes, as this person would get close enough for me to see their features clearly, I would have to make them leave. Some of these people came to me in this fashion several times before I would let them close enough to me to hold a conversation. Once I "let" them speak to me, I "gave" them the words I wanted to hear. This person would have their voice (as I remembered it) but I gave them the words. And out of their mouths came the acknowledgment that they hurt me. They would tell me how they hurt me and sometimes would tell me why. Sometimes it took several "meetings" just listening to their confessions before I let them get to asking for an apology. Then I gave them the words I needed to hear from them. And then I let them physically show me how very sorry they truly were. Some of them cried, some hung their heads in shame, others just gave me the sad confused eyes. Then, I would tell them, from the bottom of my heart, "It's done. You have my forgiveness."

I know this sounds really weird to some of you right now. But this works. It works for those who have hurt you who have since died as well.

Another "truth" came to me during this process. I believe that we will be forgiven as we learn to forgive others. I also believe that we will be judged as we judge others. Let's say, for instance, that I was sitting in judgment of my mother. And, let's say, I refused to allow her to "get off the hook" I had put her on. Now, I look at my life and all the stupid human mistakes I have made and I look at my son. Why should I ever expect to have my son "forgive" me for things I did or didn't do that he may someday blame me for if I couldn't be "woman" enough to do the same for my mother?

None of us are perfect. Each of us (unless truly psychotic) does the best we know how to do at the time. It may be the wrong thing, it might be seen to be an evil thing. But how often are we cognitive enough at the time of action to know what effects our actions or words will have on another person at that moment or years from that moment? God gave us the power and privilege to have the capacity to forgive. It is a gift left unwrapped for many of us. Unwrap this precious gift and find a way to use it. The freedom that comes to your world, the knots that get untied in the stomach are all well worth it. You also receive the extra added benefit of not wasting tremendous time and energy babbling on and on about your past to anyone who will hear you as you make an effort to be "heard" or validated in some way.

If you are no longer physically under the domain of your oppressor, let him or her go from your life. Stop playing the victim. Without the role of victim, the play has no choice but to end. You control that. You can do that.

What I have just relayed to the reader in the last few paragraphs dealing with forgiveness may come across as too simplistic and a process that can be accomplished in an afternoon. What I wrote took me nearly two years to work through. It is a grueling and tiresome ordeal. Without my being too ill to work, I might not have ever done it. Facing facts and facing buried emotions is an ordeal that you cannot harness and decide you've had enough and stop it from coming. You can't in other words, scratch the surface, deal a little, go to work and out to the world and function. That is what I had done in the past and it never worked for me. It's like opening Pandora's Box. Once it's opened, it's opened. I am, from this experience, this cleansing, a completely different person. I am grateful for the illness because it afforded me the privilege to work through this at my own pace as I was able. If I had to put on a smile and face the world each day, I may not have had the courage to attempt this. Not that it can't be done. I know many wonderful, beautiful people, who have and continue to learn these truths as their life allows. It is much harder that way, but just as (if not more so) rewarding!

As I continue to share what I have learned with who ever wants to know, I'm surprised to hear, "Oh, I read about that in "so-in-so's" book." Or, "Okay Barb, I understand. What you're describing is Zen principles." (and so on)

Truth is, I cannot give credit to my learning spiritual truths to any specific author or human lecturer. What has become, my truth, came during the times when reading was nearly impossible. When I could read, I read the Bible. I do not want you to give me credit if I've written anything here that creates growth and understanding. Credit the Source. And I need to remind you of something I have already addressed. I believe there is no such thing as "original thought."

Something else I learned that I would like to share. It is a truth that I try very hard not to forget. If I learn to accept people as they are, no preconceived expectations of what I want them to be, accepting them just as they are, then these people will have less of a chance to hurt me to the point where I find myself in the judgment seat. If I'm not judging them, what have I to forgive of them? You see, you only need to offer forgiveness to someone you have presided judgment over. Don't judge them, you don't need to forgive them. Let their judge be their Creator. Not you. Try to live that way and you'll pick up less "barnacles" on your "hull" along the way.

Reaching higher plateaus

The changing of my attitude and the continuous spiritual growth was bringing a healing from within. My life was the same, full of pain, full of limited activity, but my approach to the whole thing had changed. I turned to reading my Bible whenever the cognitive thinking allowed it. I was searching for instructions and the spiritual meat to keep me going. I found it there. I concluded at some point, "When all else fails, read the directions" and since the Bible had been presented to me in that way as a young child, it was natural for me to turn there.

I began to feel more comfortable in my prayer life. I stopped worrying whether or not I was saying the "right" thing and chose to say whatever was on my mind (nice or not so nice) and trusted that God would sort it out.

I always thought I believed in miracles. I mean, someone says they saw one or had one, how do you challenge them? And the bible is full of records of miracles, but I never once prayed for one for myself. I would have earnestly prayed at that time for a miracle for my husband or son but I couldn't bring myself to ask for one for myself. Not that I didn't believe. I was still struggling with learning how to think of myself as being "worthy" enough of a person to ask of such a thing, let alone have one given to me. With all my growth, I still had a ways to go.

One day, during a streak of the loss of cognitive thinking where I couldn't read (this one had been going on for nearly 6 weeks) I became so depressed and so angry I was in tears. I prayed to God that if He could just let me read I would undertake studies on how the body works and through that knowledge I would apply it to myself. I said to Him that I knew these drugs were not helping me and I needed to get off of them and find a natural way to bring about health, to balance myself physically. I promised if He could do that, I in return, would pass on or share in any way possible what I learn to others who were sick.

That same day, I asked Richard to get some books for me. I know he must have thought I was totally nuts. At the time I couldn't even read the funny papers and here I was asking for science books on the immune system and books on herbs and ones on alternative health approaches. But he didn't question it even though I didn't tell him (I told no one) about the prayer and about the promise. He brought those books home and I had a miracle.

From that day on, I was able to comprehend and absorb every book I picked up that had anything to do with health, diseases, treatments and so on. Not only could I comprehend and absorb it, but I could re-explain it to anyone on a level that they could understand. It was this "miracle" that opened the doors to my purpose in life. Even though I didn't know then how I would share what I learned. I just know from the bottom of my heart, that I am suppose to share what I have learned with any one who wants to hear.

During my time of study and experimenting with theories and remedies (some I thought would nearly kill me!), I could not read and comprehend anything else. I could read a book as dry as Grays Anatomy and feel as though I was reading the greatest novel ever composed, but I couldn't put the words together to read a comprehensive sentence in the newspaper. It was quite a strange life experience.

During this time I chose to begin weaning myself from all medications. I began to feel a truth. The drugs suppressed my symptoms, although not well, but they did. Each drug also had its own side effect. Some of their side effects were pretty bad. I wanted to feel right. To feel balanced. I knew that would not happen for me on the medications. (PLEASE: do not duplicate this until you are sure this is right for you.)

If you stop reading at this point and want to take with you one truth that will bring about a healing and a balance in your life, then engrave in your mind (and then act upon it) the words a fellow by the name of Paul wrote in a letter to a group called the Corinthians. It's found in the Bible in Ist Corinthians, chapter ten and it's put into verse 30. It says (in every-day words) that whatever you choose to put into your bodies, whatever you choose to do with your lives, do so all to the glory of God.

Think about that. If you believe, as I do, that we are created by God and are here to serve one another, why would you want to damage yourself - damage His creation? If you begin to make conscience choices as to what you put into your body, you will come to understand that it is stupid to put dead food in there. It is stupid to create negative thoughts and let them live in you. It is stupid to read, listen to or watch anything that is harmful to your physic or to your emotional and spiritual health.

Another way to put this. Right now, you are the sum total of everything you have ever eaten, drank, smoked, watched on TV, read in a book, words heard and spoken and so on. If you don't like the sum total of what you have become, change the input.

The following is an example of an "answer" revealed to me through writing. I was struggling with self doubt and this entire piece simply "came."

THE DANCE
Barbara Mascio

The steps were instinctive. The movement, the rhythm always known. Simply stepping both feet, one at a time, toes pointed, as my Teacher had taught me. The foot holding the wisdom of when to ground and when to slide. Each step fluid with the last and the next. Trustfully, faithfully, I danced the step.

They began to tell me that I could not dance. I did not listen. Their insistence grew and they continued to challenge me. "What right did I have to believe my stepping was a dance at all?" they chided. With conviction, they pointed to my previous steps and said, "See, some of those steps were out of time. See, some of those steps you call dancing were not even a part of the dance!"

And so, pointing my toes forward, as I and you must do to move at all, I turned my head to see the past stepping - to see which moves were out of time. My eyes searched the past. My mind focused on the judgment and I too saw the err. I began to see that I had indeed missed the beat, stepped out of time. I no longer felt the confidence of the dance.

As I turned to the past, my feet quickly became tangled, causing me to fall. I regained my posture, tipped my toes in preparation of the step, still turning my head to see the last step. I fell again. I continued to search the past step scrutinizing each one made in error and I continued to fall. After many many falls, I realized that I was no longer dancing. I was fixed. Not progressing; no longer a fluid part of the rhythm.

I laid there determined to discover the cause of my falling. I wanted to dance again, wanted to feel the rhythm, and I wanted to stop the pain I felt with each fall.

It came to me that I could not progress with the dance, exalting the rhythm, if my eyes were not facing the same direction as my toes. I wondered if this simple fact could be the reason for my falling.

I stood up, pointed my toes and began the dance. I was cautious as I did not welcome the bruising of another fall. My head, my eyes, my focus, were on one step at a time. I relinquished my feet to the rhythm, trusting my feet would know the step. I conditioned myself not to turn to look at the previous step, and conditioned myself not to be concerned with the future step. I only had the desire to live in the step of now.

Soon, sooner than I had expected, I began to dance in rhythm, with conviction. My dance was unique and beautiful.

Then they began to say, "Your dance is one of peace and love. It is a joy to watch! Please introduce me to your Teacher!"

"A man's heart deviseth his way; but the Lord directeth his steps."
Proverbs 16 vs 9

"He brought me up also out of an horrible pit, out of the miry clay, and set my feet up on a rock, and established my goings."
Psalms 40 vs 2

> *"You gain strength, courage, and confidence by every experience in which you stop to look fear in the face"*
>
> **Eleanor Roosevelt**

Chapter 5

"I promise ... through sickness and in health ..."

I asked Richard if he would share, in his own words, what it was like for him to go throughout this whole transformation with me. We were married only three years when I first started having health problems. By the time our 5th wedding anniversary came we were struggling with serious health problems and enormous financial strains as well. Becoming ill, not being able to work, was devastating on our budget. We had always tried to live within our means but when your "means" drastically changes overnight it is pretty hard to recoup.

Richard is seven years younger than I am. I feel that this is somewhat important to mention as it explains some of the heightened anxiety I was feeling in becoming, what I perceived, a burden.

So. Here is this younger man who suddenly finds himself in a marriage with a woman who cannot fulfill her needs, let alone even recognize his. A partnership where half of the earning power was now on the couch or in bed for an indefinite period of time. How did he do it? Why did he do it? Could I have done it if the roles were reversed?

I have never known human love that could transcend the true meaning of love - unconditionally. I was always mentally prepared for him to turn to me and say, "I love you, but..." He never did.

When I look back at the years I spent struggling and being so self focused on the illnesses and on the search for health, I realize I have little if no memories of what was going on in Richard's' life. He was very much alone during that time much of the time. He did ask for and receive help and strength from his family and I am so grateful that they were there for him.

He put my needs before his needs. He did this, not in the fashion of a martyr. He did it from the seat of love and I cannot explain how he did it. I don't think he can either. Not really.

Today, things are great. I'm healthier than I ever thought a person could be. We grew through this tragedy in our lives, together, not apart. We reached each step towards balance, hand in hand, together. I feel so much love and compassion for what he was put through and yes, I am grateful. I do not feel however, as though I now "owe" him or am "obligated" in any way. Richard would hate that.

We both came through this with a greater appreciation for our love, for our marriage, for one another and for having a Christian marriage where God and spirituality are very much a reality.

It would be "normal", I suppose, for Rich to lord over me now a bit. " ... after all I have done for you ..." He doesn't. I know he won't. He loves me.

We wanted to share this part of the journey with you because you need to know it is hard to go through what we did but it is possible. We both find it difficult to find the words that encompass the love and the love "actions" that developed through this trial of ours. It is so simple to say, "I love her, of course I would stick it out with her." People want to know, "Yes, but how? How exactly did you do it?"

We've both tried to answer and address this in this chapter. I hope it comes across clear enough but I know it doesn't come close to giving you a definitive answer. That is the mystery of love I suppose. Now Richard has his turn to reveal his part in all of this...

I can remember the phone call as if it were yesterday. Barb was on the phone and I could hardly hear her, all I could tell was that she needed me home and she needed me now. I told my boss something was wrong at home and I left. We lived only about 10 to 15 minutes from where I worked. When I got home I found Barb curled up in a fetal position in the empty bedroom. The headache and body pain had overwhelmed her to the point where she could only lay there. She was beginning her road to hell. We were in the process of moving because Barb had resigned from her job as a property manager. She had been unable to perform her needed tasks, at least as well as she thought she should, due to her decreasing cognitive functions. What had once been an easy task had turned into an all day project. Imagine being a painter and slowly forgetting how to blend colors, or even the names of a particular color at times. The frustration and anger was matched only by the pain and worry, and that day, Barb felt better than she would for quite some time.

Watching someone you care for as they lose the person they once were is not easy. It helps to remember that any discomfort or agitation you feel is magnified twenty-fold within the other person. As Barb's descent began, the changes were slower than toward the end. Her cognitive abilities lessened. Things that would have been no problem just a few weeks earlier now caused much effort and aggravation. As this progressed, she became more and more irritable. There can be no wonder. Imagine yourself in the same situation. If a month ago you could play improvisational guitar and now you can't even remember a C-major chord without having to look up the fingering, it would cause no small amount of concern.

One thing to remember. Never, never doubt your partner, if they are making efforts to get well. By this I mean are they keeping their doctor appointments, following their suggestions, searching for answers. If they are taking an active role in the search for their change in health, then you must believe that this is not something that they are bringing on themselves. With this being the case, you as the "well" one must support and be understanding of what your partner is going through.

Depression is something that will occur. Not a clinical-type depression but a depression brought about by the events that are occurring. There is a world of difference. Do not work with the assumption that depression is depression is depression. Imagine how you would feel if you used to play the guitar (or any instrument) and over the course of two to three months you lost the use of your hands. It is a reactionary depression.

I remember many tearful conversations as Barb would be mourning for her "old life." I internally mourned for my "old Barb." Watching as your loved one struggles with a life-changing illness is not easy. You must learn to be patient, calm, compassionate and most importantly, you must learn to ignore. Yes, ignore. Many things may be said or done that are done out of frustration or despair that you just cannot take to heart. On several occasions Barb asked for a divorce. She said "You can live here if you want but I don't want to prevent you from having a life of your own. Please divorce me." This would break my heart. She did not want a divorce because she stopped loving me, she wanted one because she loved me more than herself. How could I even consider leaving someone who (a) I loved more than anything (b) needed me for support no matter what she said and (c) loved me enough in spite of her own illness to consider my life more important than her own. Do not take this to mean that this was the easy decision. It would undoubtedly have been easier on me to pack up and go. There was no end in sight to this malady. Our social and personal lives were nonexistent. All day, every day was devoted to maintaining pain and taking care of Barb and the house. This tends to get tedious after three years. But, just like I told Barb after one of the more insistent episodes of asking me to divorce her, when I married her I did so out of love and not just convenience or to have someone to split the bills with. I vowed before God and man to love her through sickness and in health. I had had some great "healthy years" and now it was up to me to honor the vows through some sick ones. I refused to believe that it would be this way forever; it was a matter of getting to the "other side." And I wanted to be there to experience the joy of having Barb back again.

I guess I summed it up best when talking with a friend of mine a few years later when asked how I did it. I answered, "I didn't even really consider any other option. I was healthy, Barb was sick. I was not the one with the problems, not really. My goal was to help Barb get through this. I am her husband, that's what I was supposed to do, right?" He seemed amazed at my simplistic view. He said not many men would have stuck through having no sex life, let alone all the other problems, by reasoning that "the wife was not keeping up with her obligations." My answer to that is any person who places more importance on his or her own comfort than the well being of their spouse or family just wasn't paying attention when they were at the alter.

While this was happening, something even worse was happening in our lives. Our friends and family were slowly (and not so slowly) but surely stopping to come around. It would be like when someone dies and everyone begins to think , "He/She needs to get on with their life. I don't have anything else to say or do for them." These people are getting uncomfortable. They do not have the same endurance as you because they don't have to have it. They are able to go on with their "good ol' lives" and try to forget what you are going through. Actually, good for them. How many of us when faced with a chronically ill friend don't wish it would all just go away? And if this person is not among your close circle, how long do you stay or how often do you see them? Not as often as you would like to admit, I'd bet. It is uncomfortable to not be able to help. Believe me I know. But sometimes the greatest help you can give is to just not give up. Be there, let them know that you care and believe in them as a human being. It is this that is being eroded as they are unable to work or even "pitch in" around the house as they used to. These people are being stripped of their old lives and beliefs, and if you stick around you may just find someone you didn't know existed who is quite wonderful in their own right.

The love of, and for, your family and friends are the one commodity that cannot be taken from you by any municipality, government or agency. This is why I love my wife so much. I know, without doubt, that she will always love me. Just for who I am, not for what I do, what income I have, address I live at, or possessions I buy her.

My love for Barb gave me the strength to get through each day regardless of the set-backs; it was the love my family had for both of us that gave me the ability to endure. Without the support of God, my Grandma, my father and especially my mother, I would have felt very much alone and stranded. Even when all they did was listen and sympathize, they enabled me to get some of the worry out of my system. I know they shared my pain. There are not enough words in the world to tell them how much I needed them and how I was, and still am, thankful they were there for me. I am not so foolish as to realize that not all people going through this kind of ordeal have this kind of familial support. For those without family support, for any reason, you must stay focused on your loved one who is sick. Remember, they need you more than you do for now.

Another way I was able to keep sane was work and hobbies. The other employees at my shop were not aware, completely, of the turmoil at my house. Work was an escape. I would lose myself there, just to give my mind a break. My hobbies included basketball, golf and music. On the rare occasions that I could get away, I did. You should too. Your partner will be OK for a few hours. By doing this, I was able to truly be there for Barb and not be resentful or wishing I was elsewhere. If you don't have any hobbies, GET ONE. Anything. It can be as simple as needlepoint or as complex as computer building. Even if it is only once a month, you have to take time for yourself. Even an hour. Allowing your mind and body the chance to recharge for the next wave of bullshit. Because it will come and you need to be ready. At least as ready as possible.

There were many times that I wished the doctors would find something, anything, just so that we would have an answer to Barb's suffering. We actually hoped that there was a tumor at one point. At least then the enemy would have a name. The worst had to be when we went to a well respected, world-renowned hospital in Cleveland. We were told by all who knew us "Thank God, now you will certainly get an answer." Our hopes were high that something would be found. After the tests, the head neurologist walked in and calmly told us that the problems were coming from marital strife and that Barb needed only to see a clinical psychologist!! He was not even able to look us in the eye when he talked. When Barb began to cry, the only thing he could say was "See, you're over-emotional. Let me make you an appointment." He completely disregarded the fact that Barb had been in pain for the last year and a half and we were hoping beyond hope that this pinnacle of modern medicine would be able to help her, and us.

Test after test, doctor after doctor. Nothing was helping us to find the cause for Barb's dysfunctions. Meanwhile, Barb was getting more and more angry, frustrated and hopeless.

Living with someone who has CFIDS is not for the faint of heart. It takes courage, patience, love and more patience. Barb would say things from pure emotion, that even though she may have wanted to mean, didn't or couldn't. I believe this. Remember when you, the reader may have been hurt at one time and when someone came to comfort you and you said something like, "Leave me alone. I'm fine. I don't need or want your help!" But deep on the inside is a person, who even while hurting, would have cherished nothing more than to be held and told "It's going to be O.K. I'm here and will help in any way I can." Some people may see this as a sign of internal weakness.

In my opinion, if you are able to say, "This is more than I am able to handle alone. Please walk this road with me, my friend," you are stronger than Hercules.

And if you, as their friend, say in return, "I will help in any way I can. I may not understand what you are going through, but I know I love you and I am here," you are not only brave, but the very friend that your friend desperately needs. Whether they want to admit it or not.

Living and loving someone with CFIDS, or any chronic illness, is far from easy, but not impossible. Give all you can to God. He's stronger than any of us. He loves us and will give us what we need. Just ask. The answer given may not be the one you want, but you will get an answer, just quiet down enough to listen. I wanted Barb to be well the first month she was sick. It did not happen. I knew there was something more in store for us. I did not know what but I knew there was something. More than three years later I finally got the answer I was looking for. But we needed this time to grow. The lessons we learned together and alone were preparing us for a life that, while not as corporately driven, has reaped more rewarding experiences than if Barb had gotten well quickly and gotten on with our "old life." Do not be resistant to change. As blunt as this sounds, your old life is probably over. But, if you look around as you go, you will, undoubtedly, see things that perhaps, previously, you were too busy to see.

One last point I would like to make. Like one of my favorite shows, The X-Files, says, We are not alone. There are others going through the same thing you are. Find them. Contact local health professionals, hospitals, health food stores, find out if there is a CFIDS support group in your area. If there is not, start one. Just type up some flyers and leave them at health food stores, alternative health practitioners' offices, anywhere people will let you. Even if one person calls you and you can talk, that is one person more than you had before. You might even find a long-term friend. I, meanwhile, am praying for you. Any one person who opens their heart and allows their Higher Power access will find all the strength they need. Even while filled with despair, every day that goes by gets you one more day closer to the end. Just believe with all you've got that there is an end, there will be. It just might take a while. And a little work. But it's wonderful at the other end. Believe.

Written by: Richard Mascio

Chapter 6

"THE PHYSICAL WORK"

Read this chapter with an open mind. I am not asking you to trust me here. I am asking that you trust yourself.

If you are at the point with your health and well being that I reached when I began this portion of my journey, then I will assume that you are a bit nervous.

I found the necessary element for success in this endeavor was my willingness to learn how to "listen" to my own body. Each body is different. Each having it's own rhythms. Through the process of trial and error you will discover what works for you and what does not. This philosophy earmarked the difference between my taking responsibility for my health as opposed to handing is over entirely to a physician.

I believe that pharmaceutical therapy will not cure my illness. It will suppress the symptoms. With the symptoms suppressed, in other words, no longer felt, I may think I feel better. But I believe that drugs will not bring balance to my overall health.

I AM NOT ADVOCATING THAT YOU DISCONTINUE ANY MEDICATION YOU ARE CURRENTLY TAKING. I would suggest, if you are prepared to start taking more responsibility with your own health that you do get a thorough education on all your medications and their possible side effects. Nowadays, most pharmacies are happy to supply you with that information. When I reached this point, I felt it was my responsibility to discuss the current health approach using these medications with my doctor. I needed to weigh the benefits. This was my decision but PLEASE gather as much information as possible before you actually act on a decision like this.

There are a lot of great doctors out there. I found ones who would work with me in partnership and appreciated my involvement in my path to healing. If you do not have a doctor who wants your participation, change doctors.

When I made the decision that I wanted to treat my health differently from the normal usage of medications I turned to the Alternative Health field for a guide, a naturapathic physician - someone well versed in body chemistry and food chemistry. I went on a search, in other words for a different kind of professional.

What I found is this. There are good practitioners in this field, and there are some not-so-good. There are those who have great procedures and those who do not.

My insurance company, most insurance companies, do not cover natural type healing methods. Although, dollar for dollar a naturapathic physician will cost you less over all (if working an effective method) it is quite difficult to pay out of the pocket for their services. That is especially true when you are not able to work. You may hear, as I did, "Well, isn't your health worth it?"

Boy, would that would anger me. My health was worth everything, forget trying to put a monetary assessment on it. But I was not faced with the choice of whether to pay $65 for an office call and another $50 to $60 in herbs, vitamins, etc., or to buy that new Mercedes I had my eye on. I was out of work, no form of income whatsoever, and no idea when, if ever, that would change.

In fact it was that anger that brought me here, to this chapter. I realized I wasn't looking for one individual to "save" me, make me well. I wanted to learn how to make myself well. Simply replacing a mainstream physician with a non-mainstream doctor wasn't going to be my answer. My answer was found in learning how to balance my own body.

If each professional we met on this healing journey could see themselves as teachers, we the students, all of us would have the opportunity to excel with our healing. So long as the "healing" people choose to be the figure heads, the learned masters who lead you or direct you as opposed to teaching you, then optimal health on an individual basis will be thwarted.

I realize there are those out there who will always prefer to be told what and how to do it. Normally it is their faith and respect in the "authority" figure that actually brings them a level of comfort. It also allows you to hand over the responsibility of your own health to another individual. If you choose to continue in that mind-set, be careful who you willingly give this control to.

Please note that I am not trying to come across as insulting. I highly respect both the mainstream and alternative professions and the people who make them up. It takes a great deal of personal effort to accomplish their titles.

To put this in a nutshell: I no longer felt comfortable giving the responsibility of my health to any one individual. I became a student and began the painstaking course of action found in trial and error.

This chapter outlines the actual program that I developed for myself. I found these methods to be cost efficient. They are ones you can find great improvements in without ever leaving the care of your physician (alternative or mainstream). You will decide when or if to break those ties insofar as the daily maintenance of your health.

Before you begin, there are two things we must cover.

Do not be tempted to dispute or not try something simply because it sounds so simple it "couldn't" possibly work. Some of the greatest healing comes from simplicity. And remember, I searched for simplicity and searched for methods that would be easily duplicated.

I don't know how you envision the workings of your body but I would like to give you my thoughts. If you can try to envision it the way I do then the material that follows will make greater sense to you.

The body is often discussed in "parts." Like a machine. The heart this, the lungs that, the brain this, the nervous system that. Toss that thinking out. It is much too rigid and, in my humble opinion, incorrect. Our bodies are like a garden. A full blown garden with all the negative and positive workings of any good garden. We have pests, we have weeds, we have roots, stalks, stems, buds, flowering, dying,(decay) rebirth, (germination). Every plant has within it a natural immune system. We, too, have this immune system.

Years ago, before the discovery of pesticides, farmers knew how to allow their gardens to flourish with simple methods, like planting one plant near others that would repel pests from one another. Additionally, each seed of a plant that survived pests, weather, etc. was stronger than the seed before it, causing the next crop to be healthier (more fruitful) than the one previous.

We are made up of cells, each cell holding the same kind of memory that a seed holds. If our cellular structure was able to immune itself from an invading microorganism the entire cellular structure would become stronger. Just like the seeds from a garden.

I am not a chemist, pathologist or horticulturist. But doesn't it stand to reason that if we are so similar in make up to a garden that each new cell development (which happens trillions of times a day throughout your system) should be stronger than the one previous to it? This is certainly true of bacteria's. Each year, a bacteria of the same name strikes back with increased strength. Why? When we use antibiotics to kill bacteria we kill all the weaker strands. If we're very lucky, we kill them all. Usually, we've left the stronger ones to multiply at some later date.

This may not be a pleasant thought to throw in here. But consider the cockroach. The cockroach has been around since the beginning of time. We kill them, and their eggs. So why are they still here? They adapt to the poison and through the passing of cell intelligence the next brood lives with the "knowing" of how to survive the current use of bug spray. The "memory" is held within the cell wall, within the DNA somehow.

So. The body is organic in nature and as such must be nurtured much in the same way a garden is planted and maintained.

So, let's get back to our gardens. Ever plant one? Perhaps you haven't but most people have had at least one experience with a house plant. If you want your plants to grow, flower and produce what will you first want to do?

PART ONE
PREPARE THE SOIL

Our soil is found throughout our bowel ecology. The intestines and colon. It is imperative that we have healthy flora and a balance of bacteria living within our bowel ecology. Without a healthy bowel ecology, we cannot:

- Pull nutrients from our food properly
- Properly rid our systems of toxicity
- Maintain a balance of acid and alkaline

The total implications of the above did not hit me until I gave it a bit more thought. Okay, we aren't able to pull nutrients from our food. What does that mean? Simply, you are in a state of starvation. Oh, you'd never know it. I'm sure you look and feel full. Consider this:

- Do you feel exhausted from the inside out?
- Are your nerves easily rattled?
- Is your mind cloudy?
- Do you catch colds and flu easily?
- Do you have a degenerative illness? (Heart disease, diabetes, arthritis, etc.)

or

- Do you have a weight problem (over or under?)
- Do you have CFIDS or AIDS or Asthma?
- Do you have weak muscles & or bones?

and so on....

Properly rid my system of toxicity

What happens when the toxins that have made their way down to your intestines aren't disposed of through one of your elimination systems? Where does all that stuff go to?

Your digestive tract is somewhere between 35 to 40 feet long! The outside walls of this huge body part are actually quite thin. It is muscular in a similar way that a snake is muscular. Bowel movements make their way through much the same way a snake slowly digests and pushes freshly killed prey through. Without healthy flora, without strong elasticity within the tract, the process is difficult to say the least. In fact, you may have unreleased bowel movements stored within tiny pockets throughout the tract. You just weren't "healthy" enough to pass it through and now it has taken up residence.

This could stay there for years perhaps never coming out on its own accord. The more damage presented to bowels, the less "purging" action available, the more likely that you are constipated and may not even realize it.

Blood and other body fluids continue to pass through this little cesspool you have deposited there and it's nearly impossible for these fluids to not pick up bacteria growing now in these pockets. This blood of course, circulates through your entire system. From the top of your head down to your toes and everything in between.

Not a pretty picture. And this is residue (undigested food) from foods. What about the other toxicity we are exposed to from our environment?

A foreign substance (not God made) such as preservatives, pesticides, dyes, flavorings, and so on has a different type of assault all its own. The body's "cell intelligence" isn't sure what to do with toxicity such as these. The body tends to store these and other toxins such as metals in two primary centers: your liver and your fat cells. Again, blood and body fluids circulate through these areas and the entire body is tainted.

Maintain a balance of acidity & alkaline

The acid alkaline balance at the cellular level should be 80% alkaline / 20% acid. Your individual cells are what make up each organ, hemoglobin, cilia and so on. Too much alkaline and you are out of balance in a way that will make you feel washed out. Too much acid and you will have skin problems and strong smelling urine. Too much alkaline and you foster the growth of some nasty strong bacteria. Too much acid and you inhibit the growth of healthy strong bacteria. This imbalance of bacteria growth leads to illnesses of all sorts.

HOW DO YOU PREPARE THE SOIL?

Let's say you had a patch of ground that you wanted to plant vegetables in. It was overgrown with grass or weeds and since it had never been plowed, it was dense, hard. The goal is to plant the vegetables and raise them organically. The task in front of you will be time consuming. You have learned that you should begin preparing the soil ahead of the actual "planting day." This gives the ground the time it needs to "rejuvenate." Duplicating your efforts from time to time (each season to be exact) will be necessary and so you are mentally prepared for the fact that this is not a "one time" effort on your part. The prospect of juicy fresh green vegies on your familys' table inspires you on.

Remove the top layer of weeds and, as any good farmer will tell you to do, give the ground some "breathing" time. Adding some live compost (preferably from an animal whose diet has been 80% alkaline/20% acid) to feed the soil is a must. You let that work in and you see more weeds. Repeating the weeding cycle and then allowing time for your garden to soak in nutrients from the rain and the sun is a natural choice, followed by another layer of compost. Usually at this point you will add a layer of healthy nutrient rich topsoil. You give it time to assimilate. The ultimate goal is healthy vibrant soil.

This is exactly what I did with my bowel ecology. I proceeded cautiously and methodically. I was very aware of my symptoms of Malabsorption and the Irritable Bowel Syndrome. If you have ever had colon spasms, uncontrollable diarrhea or chronic constipation, you will agree with me that the last thing you want to do is to cause any irritation.

This is what I did:

WEED & FEED

1. For 7 days I took a small dosage of an herbal colon cleanser. (See Product Information)

I swallowed the capsule with a full glass of water before going to bed

SEED

2. For the next 14 days this would be the regime:

A. Upon rising I would consume 7 capsules of Acidophilus (See Product Information)

For best results, Acidophilus should be consumed on an empty stomach. You are in the most alkaline state at this time and your system will have a better chance at cultivating. You should wait 20 min. after taking it before you eat or drink anything other than water.

B. Before going to bed, I would consume 7 capsules of Bifidus with a full glass of water. (See Product Information)

For best results, this bacteria culture should be taken at night,when your system is more acid.

3. For the next 7 days I let my bowel ecology rest.

This cycle takes 28 days, just a little under a month. Marking the calendar always helped so I could remember where I was.

When the cycle has been completed once you will need to discover within your own self if you have been able to effectively accomplish your goal. The goal being to clean, weed, and plant healthy bacteria. If you no longer have colon spasms, abdominal cramping or pain, you no longer have irregular bowel movements (diarrhea or constipation) then chances are you're on the right track.

I would suggest that you continue with a maintenance program. My maintenance program is:

A. 2 Acidophilus in the morning

B. 2 Bifidus in the evening

C. 1 herbal cleanser 3 times a week (or as needed)

What is a normal bowel function? You should have a bowel movement 20 to 40 minutes after you eat a meal. You are not excreting the food you just ate, this is debris from a previous meal and you are simply making room for the food you just ate.

Be patient as this will take some time to accomplish using the conservative methods I have used.

WHAT ARE THE BENEFITS OF USING PROBIOTICS?

1. You are increasing the population of friendly bacteria. The more friendly bacteria you have, the less room for deadly bacteria.

2. Studies have shown that Acidophilus will produce non-toxic antibiotics that your immune system can put to good use. It is currently being studied for the properties it has to lower cholesterol. It addresses the health of the small intestines.

3. Bifidus addresses the health of the large intestines. It does for this area what the acidophulis does for the small intestines.

4. The herbal cleanser I use not only helps to soften your stool it also adds nutrients to your cilia.

HOW DO YOU KNOW YOU ARE ON THE RIGHT TRACK?

When you begin to have three normal (soft but whole) bowel

movements a day. When the bowel movements have little or no odor.

I have used the above cycle often. Each time I feel myself getting stronger within. Each time I have continued evidence that I am on the right track.

WHAT CAUSES THE FLORA TO BECOME DAMAGED?

Antibiotics, birth control pills, caffeine, chlorinated or fluoridated water, alcohol, processed foods, not enough raw foods, poor digestion (lack of digestive enzymes in the diet allowing whole foods to putrefy), chemical additives, ant-acids, smoking and stress are the most widely accepted culprits for the desecration of these probiotics.

I can only speak from my experience with this process and please know there are a ton of text books and other reading material available for your own studies on the subject concerning bowel ecology.

I know that some things did not work, in fact they made me feel even more weak and ill. I do not want to get into remedies that did not work. I truly want to focus on the ones that have and continue to work for me.

Experiment with this. I cannot emphasize enough how vitally important rejuvenating your bowel ecology must become for you if you have a chronic illness. You need this support system laid down firmly before much else you do will matter.

The process of attending to my pre-digestion, digestion and elimination resulted in my finally being capable of consuming raw fruits and vegetables. I now have healthy bowel movements and no longer suffer from colon spasms. Additionally - my weight has begun to balance.

If you do not work on this area first, many of your other efforts will fail. Not because they are incorrect efforts, but because your body is not healthy enough to assimilate them.

TEND TO YOUR SOIL !!!

CAUTION !!!

When I was in the middle of full symptoms and in a weakened state, the above regime had to be altered! It was imperative that I proceeded with caution. Trust that the body has the wisdom to know if it is capable of "detoxifying" in this manner and it will send definite signals to let you know if you are causing more harm than good. The following is how I began to bring life to my elimination system, while in a weakened state and in full symptoms:

Rather than "clean & weed" first I needed to add the "seeds" in the beginning. This allowed me to have the strength and the "health" required to follow through with the "cleaning" and the "weeding."

THE CAUTIOUS METHOD

FEED

1. For 14 days:

2 Acidophilus upon rising (again with a full glass of water and wait 20 minutes before eating or drinking anything but water)

2 Bifidus before going to bed, with a full glass of water.

2. Each week that follows:

I increased the Acidophilus and the Bifidus by one each week until I was able to consume 7 at a time with no ill side effects. This took another 5 weeks (35 days)

3. For 2 weeks:

7 Acidophulis in the morning

7 Bifidus in the evening

WEED & SEED

4. For 7 days:

1 herbal colon cleanser in the evening

5. Next 14 days:

Rest, do nothing

6. Maintenance:

2 Acidohpulis in the morning

2 Bifidus in the evening

1 herbal colon cleaner once a week

This plan takes longer but achieved the results I was looking for in a slow methodical fashion without risking a shock to my system that I did not want to endure at the time. I repeated the cycle as often as I felt I needed to. The body will send you the signals to let you know if you are in need of another "weeding" or "planting."

Some products worked for me and some did not. Often times it wasn't the product itself, it was how the company who manufactured and processed it that made the difference. If you would like to purchase the same products I use please refer to the phone numbers listed in the back of this book. With probiotics you want "live" bacteria. One hint, if it doesn't require refrigeration, it is not "live." Some companies, in order to deliver a less costly product, will use heat during their manufacturing process. Heat kills enzymatic action and will kill the bacteria. So, even if the label lists all of what you are looking for, you need to find out how the finished product is manufactured. This can be nearly impossible with some companies, while others are more than happy to send you the information you are requesting. The fact that I will recommend specific companies is only because I have found them to be extremely conscientious in their choices in manufacturing and harvesting. I am not saying that there are not other companies out there who are just as good or perhaps even better. (?)

Again, this is your journey, your experimentation. I am only sharing what I have learned and what has worked for me.

PART TWO
BASIC FUNCTIONS of the ELIMINATION SYSTEM and the LYMPHATIC SYSTEM

This section will explain in simplistic terms a bit of information on how our bodies work. Again, I emphasize I am not a physician, I am a student. I am relaying what I came to regard as pertinent knowledge to help me understand what was going on inside this body of mine.

Your body has as one of it's functions, an elimination system. It is intricate and interrelated. If each elimination juncture is not working properly, you will not have the ability to rid yourself of past toxicity still hanging around, let alone the current toxicity that daily bombards your system. Once you understand how these systems work then you will appreciate the need to discontinue current daily habits that are insulting the system. If you are ill now you have quite a bit of toxicity to rid yourself of. Why compound the problem by adding daily doses?

Each area has a specific job but each area depends on one

anothers cooperation. If, for example, you are not able to rid your-self of a toxin in the colon, the body fluids carry that toxic residue along . One body fluid is blood, another, lymph fluid. Lymph fluid flows through the lymphatic system into lymph nodes. Lymph nodes are special sites in the body that act as filtering stations. They also (when working properly & not overly taxed with poi-sons) are the manufacturers of lymphocytes. Lymphocytes are what help us protect ourselves from invading organisms; viruses and harmful bacteria. The task of these nodes is to ensure that once toxicity comes to it, it filters it as free of poison as possible before it releases it back out into the blood stream. There are over 600 lymph nodes in the body all in specific positions. (There are over 150 of them in the neck region alone!)

Swollen glands, soreness in the neck and throat, soreness and pain in your joints, for long periods of time, indicate the lymphat-ic system is in overload. If all its energy is being spent on detoxi-fying it will have less energy to produce the lymphocytes we need in our army of defense.

And so the problem of toxicity must be looked at as being "cir-cular." I (in my humble opinion) cannot believe that you can "detoxify" your liver and not be prepared for that toxicity to leave the liver and end up in some other place within the body.

Personal Story:

I went to an herbalist once who suggested I consume a variety of cleansing type herbs. He had no doubt that I was brimming with toxins. I had to agree. And he was right. I was. The problem was that very little, of any, of my elimination systems were func-tioning efficiently. By taking in de-toxifying herbs with no regard to "how" those toxins were going to get out once released, I had a horrific reaction. My skin turned a pale yellow, the whites of my eyes were yellow, the palms of my hands were nearly orange. I was extremely ill. I began with stomach nausea and constipation. This soon let lose into days of diarrhea.

What happened? He was right. I was full of toxicity. He was right. I needed to de-toxify. He was correct in his choosing of herbs, in that his choice in herbs was cleansing herbs. What he did-n't take into consideration was that I FIRST needed to attend to strengthening my elimination systems.

So please do not attempt a full body cleansing if your elimination systems are not working. Otherwise you will stir up this toxin and it will recirculate with no way of getting out.

There are health clinics and spas that are structured to monitor and assist you through a cleansing process. They will include (among other things) massage, water therapy, diet, colonics, saunas, and so on. They are staffed with professionals who will medically attend to you while you go through this much needed healing crisis.

I could not afford to attend one. My insurance would not cover it and I did not have the funds. I believe that it would have been extremely beneficial and would have sped up my recovery. This was not possible for me and so I had to find other ways. If you are financially capable, check them out.

PART THREE
THE CELLULAR LEVEL

Every minute part of who you are is found in the individual cellular makeup. Each cell is a tiny universe within itself. A healthy cell is 80% alkaline / 20% acid. Cells split and make new cells. Cells die and other cells take care of the debris from the dead cells. Cells generate electrical energy connecting the "dialect" between one area of the body to another.

Each cell contains "blueprints" of who you are and who all your blood relatives are in the form of DNA. This is the reason behind your being "predisposed" for certain degenerative illnesses.

Each cell also holds within itself actual memory. Each cell recording within it not only physical information but emotional information. As the cell dies it passes all this accumulated information on to the new replacement cell.

Let that last paragraph sit with you for a minute.

Consider the implications. Know this. Optimum health cannot be achieved through addressing one avenue of your being. You are Spirit. You are Mind. You are Body. You are Energy. All this is you. To address your health with focused vision on one aspect will be ineffective.

And so, you will see as you continue here that this journey towards "health" is not found in discovering a cure. Rather, you are seeking the balance within and without your very being.

You could study cells for years and never have their full knowledge as science is constantly discovering more information. What I have touched on is about on the level and context of a grade school science text-book. It is much more complicated but if you can just put the basic idea in your mind how vitally important the health of your tiny little cells are in relationship to your whole being, it is enough to grasp the importance of what to do to assist those cells to grow, to eliminate, to de-toxify and to regenerate.

There are many factors that assist cellular health. There are just as many that interfere with the health of the cell. We can do a great deal on our own to aid the life of the cell.

It is the law of nature to survive. Each cell wants to survive. That is wonderful, so long as you are talking about a healthy cell. It is deadly if you are talking about a cancerous cell.

The Greek philosopher Heraclitus once said, "You cannot step into the same river twice." Why? A river is constantly being changed with new water moving through it at all times. Our spirit, our mind, our body, our energy is the same. It is constantly changing. The fact that cells die and are immediately replaced with new ones prove that.

For example, did you know that your skin is completely replaced within a period of thirty days? Your stomach lining is new every four days? The liver is brand new every six weeks?

Why. Why are we not healthier with each cell replacement? It has to be related to one of two answers, in my opinion.

One. The replacement cell is "born" inheriting the same qualities and the same defects of the cell it came to replace.

Two. We have inadvertently damaged a healthy cell with toxicity. Which then cycles into answer number one.

The solution then is to : One: Change or alter the cell that is about to cycle (or die) so that its cell memory can reach a healthier plateau before it passes it on to the replacement cell. Two: Stop toxifying ourselves with new assaults.

Food, environmental poisonings, drugs, and so on are obvious culprits of toxicity. Keep in mind we are addressing our health as a whole which includes your mind and spirit. These encompass your emotions, your belief systems , your thoughts.

We have all heard, "You are what you eat." Remember the other old saying, "You are what you think you are."

Just as we have discussed, optimum health is found when you combine the spirit/mind/body. The same holds true when reaching for optimum health of each individual cell. Each individual cell is a combination of spirit/mind/body. This chapter begins to address the importance of healing on the physical plane (body) of the cells. However;

All elements must be addressed or the healing will have limitations.

Our cells need fuel. This is provided to us in the form of food. It matters not if you are a meat-eater or a non-meat-eater, all food originates in the form of plants.

"I don't eat vegetables or fruits!" My friend Mary once said to me. And she did avoid them. She did however eat cooked vegetables and did drink juice. She was a 3 time a day meat-eater. She did accompany her meat with cooked vegetables, rice and other processed foods. The meat she consumed came from animals who ate greens and grains. Without the greens and grains, the animals she ate would not exist. (We do not eat the meat from animals who are also meat-eaters. We only eat the meat from animals who are grain eaters.) So, Mary has the exact same dilemma as those of us who rely solely on the nutrient basis of the plants we eat. No one on this planet can escape the fact that we depend on plants to survive.

I made this statement once to a group and someone spoke up, they had found a "loop-hole" in my statement. "What about fish eaters? Fish don't eat grains!"

No. But fish eat greens. Fish eat algae and fish consume the minerals from their home environment, whether that be fresh water, spring water or salt water. It is the minerals that we are after in our food.

Minerals are the tools needed to produce Vitamins. Without the proper concentration, the proper combinations of minerals, you cannot expect any living thing to produce within itself, vitamins.

WHAT ARE VITAMINS EXACTLY?

Vitamins are ORGANIC molecules, necessary in TRACE AMOUNTS, that act as catalysts in the normal metabolic processes in the body.

Unlike the "nutrients"; proteins, fats and carbohydrates, vitamins, by themselves, DO NOT provide energy. They DO NOT serve as building material either.

Most vitamins cannot be produced by the body and so must be found in our food supply. The vitamins that can be produced by the body can do so only if the provitamins are provided (again from our food supply). An example of this would be the vitamin "A." Vitamin "A" can be produced by the body only if the provitamin, a chemical know as "Carotene" has been provided. Carotene can be found in carrots or spinach for example. Another example would be that of vitamin "K" which is produced in the gastrointestinal tract by healthy bacteria in the bowel ecology.

WHAT DO VITAMINS DO?

Vitamins are basically regulatory substances that are essential in the digestion of fats, proteins and carbohydrates. Vitamins are involved IN EVERY BIOCHEMICAL ACTION IN THE BODY! Vitamins, along with minerals and amino acids, control cell respiration and are ESSENTIAL TO MAINTAINING LIFE.

There are two types of vitamins: fat-soluble and water-soluble.

The functions of fat soluble vitamins include: synthesis of glycogen; synthesis of hormones; synthesis of RNA; cartilage formation; protein metabolism in the liver; repair growth of cell membranes; maintenance of the reproductive system; and acting as coenzymes (such as Co-Q10) in the retina, bones, skin, liver and adrenal glands.

The functions of water-soluble vitamins include: tissue repair and growth; maintenance of muscle; nerve, heart and digestive tissues; synthesis of the neurotransmitter acetylcholine; acting as an essential coenzyme in all cells (important in the process of releasing energy from carbohydrates); and acting as a coenzyme in the function of the liver.

The solution then, can be found in the absolute need for our diets to consist mainly of WHOLE FOODS.

We should eat more fruits, vegetables and grains. However, it is difficult (if not impossible) to get all our necessary nutrients from fruits and vegetables.

It is almost impossible to find fresh foods that have:

•The necessary nutrient combinations

•Product that has not been saturated in pesticides, insecticides, DDT, etc.

•Product that has been raised in a topsoil medium - rich in minerals

•Product that still contain "live" Enzymatic action (not a long shelf life)

Fifty years ago one serving of spinach would give you the same amount of iron that today you would need 20 servings of. Why? 50 years ago the earth average of topsoil was 80 inches. Today, it is 8 inches. This indicates the problem we face with the loss of minerals. Remember, minerals are what help create vitamins. Topsoil is made up of minerals.

Prior to World War II there were no deadly pesticides and herbicides. These products were developed during the war and experimented with during the war. When the war was over, they had a surplus of these (and other chemicals) and looked for a way to "put them to good use" (continue to profit from their manufacture and sale). These people turned to the farming industry and "sponsored" the use of them. At first, the farmers saw wonderful results. They had less crop damage due to "pests", their crops were bigger, greener, and overall, more abundant. But when a few years had passed and their livestock (who naturally consumed the grains grown under the influence of these chemicals) began having health problems, the farmers complained. Their livestock suffered from poor growth, infertility, infections and so on. Their complaints were heard and a solution was provided. Antibiotics

& growth hormones became the common daily diet of all farm-fed livestock.

If you eat meat, you also eat what they eat. You will also consume into your body antibiotics and growth hormones.

THE NECESSITY FOR WHOLE FOODS IN OUR DIET

Without food, we slowly die of starvation. Without the necessary digestive enzymes in our diets, we cannot assimilate the foods we introduce into our bodies.

One way to make digestive enzymes work for us is in chewing. Do you chew your food long enough in order for it to be liquefied BEFORE swallowing?

If not, you are among the majority of the population.

Whole food, pieces of food, swallowed, gets dumped down through the esophagus. From there it gets dumped into the stomach. The stomach now needs to complete the process of "liquefying" your consumed food. It must do this in order to pass it through to the small intestines.

Please note: You can chew all day long and you will not create digestive enzymes from a cooked or processed food. The chemical reaction necessary comes from raw foods in combination with the saliva in your mouth.

Does your diet consist entirely of raw fresh foods? Again, if the answer is no, you are in the majority.

What will your body do then, if the necessary predigestion stage has been bypassed and digestive enzymes were not manufactured? Your body is full of enzymes - each having specific duties. Some of these enzymes are stored in major organs. When the body is signaled that digestive enzymes are needed, it will use its store house of other enzymes.

This means your body becomes dependent on using energy from major organs to digest your food. This obviously puts unnecessary stress on these organs.

Before going further, what is the definition of a digestive enzyme?

Digestive enzymes are "machines" made of protein that make chemical reactions happen rapidly enough to support life.

Without enzymes we die. Reduced digestive enzyme activity limits our ability to obtain all the necessary nutrients from our food.

The benefits to the body include (but are not limited to):

• Unlocks the nutrients in food

• Breaks down all types of foods including: protein, starch, fat, lactose and fiber.

• Aids in ridding the cells of indigestible toxins such as: preservatives coloring, chemicals, pesticides and so on.

DID YOU KNOW?

Of all the activities you could subject your body to, whether it be aerobics, running, what have you, the process of digesting food, expends the MOST ENERGY from your system? When I learned this fact, I sat up and listened. Here I was with Chronic Fatigue and through my reading I came across this tidbit of information. Learning how to manage your energy is part of this illness. If I could cause the simple repetitive action of eating to be less strenuous, less energy taxing, then I wanted to learn how. This made a great deal of sense to me.

HOW TO GET DIGESTIVE ENZYMES INTO YOUR DIET

Digestive enzyme supplements were my choice after much trial and error. There are different kinds of digestive enzymes and I wanted to keep the whole thing simple. So I found one digestive enzyme supplement that could handle all foods; protein, starch, fat, lactose and fiber. All in one capsule.

I consume 2 digestive enzymes immediately before I eat anything. This has taken the "load" off my major organs and aids my stomach in reaching the final product of liquefaction.

I recommend a specific enzyme. I've tried many others and this is the one I feel gives me the best results.

Should you decide to experiment with another brand, there are a few things to keep in mind. Many enzyme supplements address one specific element. An example of that would be to take an enzyme to aid in the digestion of dairy. This enzyme would aid typically in the breakdown of lactose but would lack the necessary element to break down the protein in the milk.

And what about the ability to aid in ridding the body of "indigestible" toxins? The enzymes act like little "pack-mans" running around and "eating" these kinds of toxins.

As mentioned before, toxins are typically stored in either the fat cells or the liver. Pesticides are a known toxin to take up residency in tissue. The use of a full spectrum digestive enzyme will go a long way in reducing your storehouse of this and other toxicities.

This, I believe, was a primary factor in my eleviation of the stiffness and pain associated with fibromyalgia within my body. Try it, and see if this helps you as well.

A KITCHEN EXPERIMENT

Make one bowl of oatmeal. Divide the oatmeal into two bowls. In one bowl, stir in 2 digestive enzymes, mix well. Set both bowls on your counter and wait about 15 minutes. Look what happened. The bowl of oatmeal with no enzymes, is thick and hard. The bowl with the enzymes is liquid enough to drink it! Is that cool or what!

This experiment convinced me of the value of digestive enzymes and how they liquefy food and aid in the predigestive process.

SO, WHAT SHOULD I BE EATING?

When you suffer from an autoimmune illness, you typically have food sensitivities. You also tend to have "cravings." Both symptoms are signs that you may have an allergy to those foods.

A pure vegetarian diet or fruitarian diet would be ideal. Especially if you can buy organically-grown produce. Although, balancing those kinds of diets can be difficult and somewhat confusing. I recommend taking a cooking class or studying cookbooks and experimenting with these diets. It can be done. You need to be concerned about minerals, vitamins, trace elements, carbohydrates, protein and amino acids. We need the full gambit to nourish us.

I am not a nutritionist and so will not recommend one specific diet over another. Each "body" has its specific requirements and working directly with a nutritionist can be very helpful.

Again, I came to this point in my healing and I could not afford to pay for a nutritionist. I was very confused about what to eat, what not to eat, when to eat, when not to eat and so on. I held fast that there had to be a whole food out there on this planet that could deliver - in a simplified manner - the balance of nutrients and proteins that my body was starving for. Again, after much trial and error and after a great deal of "searching" I "found" a whole nutrient dense food. This food grows in one place in the whole world, Klamath Lake, Oregon. It grows naturally without the aid of mankind. It is the most natural whole food on this planet.

This food is called, blue green algae. (It has also been called blue-green manna). It possesses the characteristics of all three kingdoms of life: plant, animal and bacteria.

Plant: It is able to photosynthesize and produce chlorophyll

Animal: Same digestible nutritive cell wall composed of a starch our bodies use as food

Bacteria: Same phenomenal adaptability and the ability to freely exchange genetic information and knowledge.

This was the first food that I could consume and "feel" a positive difference in my body. My sleep patterns became normal after about a month of eating this food. I finally was capable of the kind of sleep that, upon awakening, you feel "refreshed." During that first month, I also required less and less the 2 hour afternoon nap I had become accustomed to needing until I finally no longer required them at all.

I had begun the use of the digestive enzymes and the probiotics (described previously) at the same time I started with this blue green algae. As a complete food combination, addressing all parts of my body and my brain - my body responded as though it was being given a chance at re-birth. I could picture how "happy" my cells were to finally get the fuel they needed in order to perform their functions the way they were designed.

My cognitive thinking became more and more consistent. I no longer suffer any of those "down" times.

My energy level increased. Now don't misunderstand me. I don't have a "speedy" kind of energy. I have a calm sustainable level of energy that I have never known before.

Because it has the properties to nourish both the physical and mental (brain & neurological system) my attitude, my moods, my view on life in general began this wonderful healing. I am actually symptom free of PMS, something I had suffered with since I was 16 years old!

One of the most remarkable blessings I experienced was that slowly, over the course of 6 months, the pain I had become accustomed to living with, dissipated. The pain of Fibroymalgia left my body in the reverse order of how it originally manifested itself. My right elbow - the first painful spot - was the last to release the pain. In fact, with the writing of this chapter, I have been consuming the blue green algae since March of 1995 and have not suffered from any real pains anywhere in my body.

Why did this food work for me in such a noticeable manner? I really do not know, but it did!

I could quote all kinds of written material on the benefits derived from this natural food. I am not a nutritionist, chemist or physician. I cannot give you "medical" proof that it works. It is said that this food is somewhere around 97% assimilated. Your cells will recognize this as food, and since there are no additives whatsoever in it, will grab on to this food and make it work for you. This food is the most important food I can put on my grocery list, the most important food I can give to myself and to my family. Consuming as little as 3 grams a day has changed so much for me! This is the only food I eat that I know beyond all doubt has no preservatives, chemicals, and has "live" enzymatic action because of the way it is harvested and processed. I cannot say the same thing about anything else I eat.

I first began consuming this whole food in this manner:

500 mg of the algae each day for one week. Each week after I would increase the amount. I continued this until I got to where I am right now. I consume 3 grams of this beneficial food every day!

The blue green algae harvested from the company I choose to purchase it from comes in two forms. One form is the whole plant and is especially beneficial to the body and energy. The second form is the same algae except the cell wall has been deliberately "washed" away allowing better assimilation into the "brain blood barrier." This part of the food feeds the brain and neurological system among other things, like the higher functioning glands; the pituitary, pineal, thymus and so on.

These food products are available in easy to swallow caps, tablets or in the powder form. It took the mystery out of "how" to get nutrients into my body.

It is a wonderful foundation and allows me more time to experiment with the chemistry of other available foods.

In the many books written on C.F.I.D.S. and other autoimmune illnesses, vitamin, mineral and amino acid therapies are suggested and outlined. Nearly all protocol requires the expertise of a physician and most include I.V. drips. These are extremely costly (from my point of view) and most insurances won't cover them as it is considered "vitamin therapy." What excited me was I could get the suggested nutrients in the same levels for one tenth of the cost simply by consuming the blue green algae!

Is this the only food I eat? No, of course not. I eat an abundance of fresh fruits and vegetables now, along with a wide variety of grains, legumes and occasionally, chicken or fish. I no longer eat red meat or pork. I try to follow basic guidelines of ingesting a balance of 80% alkaline/ 20% acid. The following is a short but comprehensive list of both alkaline and acid foods. (The algae, by the way, is naturally 80% alkaline, 20% acid)

ACID-PRODUCING FOODS

Animal Fats	Cane sugars
Vegetable oils (all man-made oils)	Alcohol
	Artificial additives
Egg whites	Plums
Legumes	Beef
Nuts (except almonds)	Pork
White flour/ all products with white flour such as pasta	Cranberries
Starches	Animal organs
Chocolate	Caffeine (all forms)

ALKALINE-PRODUCING FOODS

Dairy products (especially from goats)

Fruits (except plums)

Vegetables (except legumes)

Seafood (except bottom feeders: shrimp, clams, oysters, lobsters, carp)

Poultry

Sunflower seeds

Almonds

Hard grains (wheat, rye, etc.)

Honey

Maple syrup (pure)

Egg yolk

Raisins

Granola

Herbal teas

I must mention a major consideration in regards to the consumption of a primarily raw diet. It truly is the best for us, however, if you experience discomfort and/or pain due to the bowel ecology being in an unbalanced state, don't push yourself. This is the reason why I began this section, many pages ago, with the absolute need to first begin there. I truly did not ever believe that I was ever going to be capable of eating this healthy way, doomed to only eating very cooked foods. I now enjoy fruits and vegetables on a daily basis! It is because I use the "Weed, Feed, Seed" and I eat my digestive enzymes before consuming food.

What is so delightful about consuming blue-green algae is that you can begin to give your body a wide variety of vitamins and minerals (etc.) right now, even before your system is capable of digesting other green whole foods!

The bottom line. I know that my body is a living organic matter. To flourish I must give it substance containing a life force. Blue-green algae and food choices that are full of life make up my diet.

To order the particular brand of blue-green algae that I use: see the back of this book!

PART IV

WATER

How important is water? Ever since 5th grade science class we've been told to drink 8 glasses a day. How many of us truly do that? By the way, 8 glasses of fluid; coffee, tea, juice and so on, do not count.

We now know that a minimum of 8 to 10 glasses of water is necessary for the person who performs no real activity. Add a walk, a fever, a plane or car trip, or a game of golf to your day and you will need to increase your water intake.

Why does the body need water? If you weigh 150 pounds, 95 pounds of that weight will constitute the weight of the water in you. More than 1/2 of the human body weight, is water. Water is contained in the blood, lymph, cells and intercellular spaces of the body. Protein and stored fat account for a further 50 pounds and the rest is glycogen, minerals and other substances, such as nucleic acids.

Every day the average person should drink an average of 5 pints of water. Keeping balance in mind, the average person will lose 5 pints of fluid every day. One pint is lost as water vapor in the breath, one pint in perspiration and three pints in urine.

Those who are struggling with their weight may find it useful to know that water may be the most important catalyst in losing weight and keeping it off. Water suppresses the appetite naturally and helps the body metabolize stored fat. Studies have shown that a decrease in water intake will cause fat deposits to increase, while an increase in water intake can actually replace fat deposits.

The kidneys cannot function properly without enough water. When they do not work to capacity, some of their load is dumped onto the liver. This causes one of the liver's primary functions (to metabolize stored fat into usable energy) to become less effective as it is now devoting much of its energy to compensate for the lack of kidney activity.

Drinking enough water is the best remedy for fluid retention. When the body gets less water, it believes that a threat to survival is happening. This signals the body to "retain" what it has.

Water also helps to maintain proper muscle tone by giving muscles their natural ability to contract and by preventing dehydration.

Water, of course, helps rid the body of waste. Enough water in your system goes a long way to aid the entire elimination system.

When your body is deprived of water, you may even suffer from constipation. With low water levels, the body siphons what it needs from internal sources. The colon is one primary source. This leads to constipation because now the colon is lacking the necessary fluids to work efficiently.

Too little water causes your body to not be able to function properly on all levels. Digestion, circulation, the endocrine gland functions, fat metabolism, maintaining balanced body temperature and so on.

Okay. What kind of water should I drink? That is a good question. I am not an authority on water supply or on water treatment devices. This is a subject for in-depth study.

What I have come to respect is the amount of bacteria and man-made chemicals in my city water supply. I have not purchased a water treatment device as of yet and so cannot recommend one personally. I have chosen; however, to purchase my water. I buy bottled drinking water. The kind I buy has been "cleaned" using what is call "reverse osmosis." This kills bacteria not necessary for consumption and yet leaves needed nutrients.

Your skin will absorb more water during a shower or bath than what you drink and so it makes a great deal of sense to have your water treated in your home to avoid the chemicals and bacteria, especially if your immune system has been compromised.

I rarely drank water before I understood the importance of it. I was a coffee and a tea drinker. I drink at least 2 quarts of water a day now and if I feel any sluggishness or stiffness in my body, I will increase that. Water is one of the best body purifiers you can consume.

If you find a source of water that tastes good, you will naturally drink more and more of it. It is one of the least expensive "foods" you can give to yourself.

You cannot function without it.

PART V
OXYGEN

Breathing is essential. You will die without breath. You can die slowly if the oxygen level is deprived or you can die rather quickly if someone pushes a pillow over your head and stops oxygen suddenly.

You know that, right? We all know that. I mean we breathe, you and I, every second or so, and have since the day the umbilical cord was cut. We don't have to "think" about it. It's just one of those body functions that happen, like how our blood pumps through the heart. That's constantly happening and we don't have any control over it. It just works. So what are you going to tell me about breathing that I don't already know?

Breathing does occur naturally and without effort or manipulation on our part. But the truth of the matter is few of us know that we can alter and change the way we breathe to benefit the entire body. We can learn how to breathe correctly.

How can you possibly breathe "wrong" you may ask. Where are you breathing from now as you are reading this. Are you breathing from your nose or your mouth? When you sleep at night, nose or mouth? As you are breathing right now, is your tummy relaxed? Is it moving with your breaths, in and out? Or is your top part of your chest breathing up and down?

Nose or mouth breathing? The nose is designed with filters for clearing the larger particles of dust from the air as it heads toward the lungs. Your mouth is not designed to filter this or any other toxic material from the air as it is mainly designed as an entrance for foods only.

For every in breath there is of course an out breath. These two kinds of breaths form in the nose creating a healthy climate. Moisture is deposited by the out breath on the mucus blanket and this is picked up by the entering in breath. The in breath grows warmer and more moist as it travels through the nose canal regulating the temperature of the air you originally breathed in. This is the reason we, as humans, can breathe in from any climate and our bodies can make use of it.

As you breathe in air, your body converts it to oxygen. There is a by-product of oxygen also produced, called carbon dioxide. The red blood cells carry oxygen from the lungs to the heart to be pumped around the body while the carbon dioxide is dispersed with your out breath.

After the oxygen has been used up, it makes its way back to the lungs to be dispersed also on the out breath. This "exhaust" is made up of 14% oxygen, 69% nitrogen, 5% carbon dioxide and the remainder percentages are made up of other toxic chemicals left behind as residue from "burning" or "using" oxygen. If you are not breathing out efficiently, it is these poisons that will eventually aid in the breaking down of your system.

The medulla (located in the brain) is responsible for the tone and diameter of the arteries. This center is sensitive to changes in the quality of the blood circulating through it. If the medulla reads an imbalance of oxygen and carbon dioxide in the blood, it reacts. This reaction could lead to a change in blood pressure, either causing it to be high or low depending on the balance.

This, I thought was quite interesting. Those diagnosed with Chronic Fatigue Syndrome are often diagnosed with low blood pressure. We typically also have low body temperatures. The illness, as well as so many other immune deficiencies or chronic illnesses, discourage any type of exercise. It is usually much too painful and in the case of Chronic Fatigue, can actually throw you into symptoms lasting for weeks. I thought this was fascinating and although I was not healthy enough at that point to begin any kind of aerobic training to correct the oxygen/carbon dioxide balance, I was convinced that learning how to alter my breathing could very well make a difference in my health. I was right. Please continue reading.

At the top of your lungs, where most of us have begun to breathe nearly all our breaths, the rate of blood flow is less than a tenth of a liter per minute. The blood flow at the bottom of your lungs, down toward the bottom of your rib cage is well over a liter per minute. Most of the blood circulation is in the bottom third of the lungs. Once you have corrected your breathing pattern your breath rate will usually drop from 14 to 15 breaths per minute to 8 to 12 breaths per minute. This is because you are getting more deeply oxygenated so that your lungs don't have to work as hard. Your heart rate will slow also, because it does not have to pump as much blood to get a full supply of oxygen to the body.

When you breathe, you need to learn how to use your

diaphragm correctly. The diaphragm is shaped kind of like a dome or a bell. It is located between the bottom of the lungs and the top of the abdomen. When you breathe in (correctly) the dome flattens. This causes your belly to expand with the in breath. When your belly expands like this, with each in breath, the vital organs get room to move and circulate more freely. You are "massaging" the organs.

When you breathe out (correctly) the dome (diaphragm) returns to its dome or bell shape. This causes your belly to contract. Again, providing a much needed massage for those internal organs.

Breathing from the bottom of the lungs in this manner as opposed to breathing shallow at the top creates more oxygen for your blood and allows the elimination of poisonous gasses like carbon dioxide to leave the body. This oxygen is life to the blood, life to each and every body cell and brain cell.

There are a lot of good books and instructors out there who can work with you one on one to teach you how to breathe correctly. This "art," if you will, goes under a few headings that may seem peculiar at first. It can be called, Yoga Breathing, Conscious Breathing, Re-Birthing, Breathwork, and so on. I highly recommend you check into it.

There are quite a few good books that also educate and instruct you on specific breathing techniques as well.

I had almost instinctively used this kind of "conscious breathing" before I knew it had a name. I had taken Lamaze class some 15 years ago and was first introduced to a form of breathing that helped you work through pain. When I became ill and was trying to live with crescendoing pain throughout my body, I found myself using some of the breathing techniques I had long since buried in my memory banks.

If you have ever given birth without the use of meds you know how beneficial it is to "breathe" into the pain.

This brings up another subject in itself. There are many books dealing with the issue of pain. Many of them ask that you visualize an ocean or some other pain-less scene in your mind and ask that you put yourself there. I have often wondered if that was indeed the best solution. I have experimented with it and with another theory who for the life of me I cannot give credit to because I do not know where I read about it. The theory is to admit you are in pain. Why lie to yourself? But then to take it further and actually breathe into the pain.

Pretend that all of your pain is held in the flame of this huge candle just out of reach of your breath. You know that if you breathe deeply and calmly enough that your out breath will be more voluminous. This larger volume of out breath will eventually blow out the flame which holds your pain. If the pain is in your eyes, breathe into your eyes in your mind. If the pain is in your colon, breathe (in your mind) into your colon.

I cannot effectively teach you how to breathe in this book. I am not that illustrative. Please follow through with this line of research on your own. The only reminder or hint if you will, that I will put here is the following:

Oxygen is vital and yet in the course of making oxygen, our bodies also makes toxic chemicals such as carbon dioxide. You need as much oxygen as you can get and you need to rid yourself of the carbon dioxide as quickly as possible.

Relax your belly (best to first start practicing lying down) and put into your mind that with your in breath you will allow your tummy to go up (out) and flatten the top of your diaphragm. With every out breath you will allow your belly to contract in pushing the diaphragm up into its original shape, the dome. Start by practicing this one breathing exercise every day for 15 minutes. You will become a believer, as I have and will want to learn more.

Another exercise I have learned to use especially if I am feeling stressed out is called alternative breathing. You use your fingers to push in one side of your nostril. While closed you breathe in (as described in the above paragraph) and when you are ready to breathe out, you release that side and close the other.

I hope I'm explaining this correctly. What you are doing is breathing in one nostril and on that out breath you release it through the other. You continue with this in out alternating between the nostrils (remember one nostril breathes in the other breathes out then switch and repeat only doing the opposite.) again for about 15 minutes every day. It will do amazing things for you!

Continue to experiment. You can practice for longer periods of time if you like. There may be times where during your breathing, out of no where, a knot will form in some place in your body. When that happens, it is a very good thing! Continue to breathe just as slowly just as methodically and focus on breathing through that knot of pain. The release that you will experience will prove to you over and over again that there definitely is something to this kind of exercise!

And now I see with eye serene,
the very pulse of the machine.
A being breathing thoughtful breath,
A traveler between life and death.

William Wordsworth

PART VI

BODY MOVEMENT

Exercise? How in the world can any one expect me to exercise when I feel so bad? I can barely make it to the bathroom and back to the bed again.

Sound familiar? It is not the voice of laziness. It is the voice of truth. No one can truly begin an exercise program in that state.

I purposely put this portion of the "work" at the end. Exercise was the last thing I personally addressed and for good reason. I could not endure the pain nor could I endure the side-effects from the exercise which if I wasn't already down would have most certainly put me down.

I was able to begin an active "BODY MOVEMENT" program on a regular basis only after I had applied the first portions of this book. I was not capable of enduring any of the stress (although good stress) that exercise would bring to the body until I was no longer in a state of starvation.

The first chapters of this book address that fairly well. You are in a state of starvation if you do not have: nutrients, minerals, amino acids, (and so on), if you do not have a healthy bowel ecology, if you do not have the balance of carbon dioxide and oxygen, if you do not have the balance of water, or if your emotional, spiritual and creative health are starving. I strongly suggest that you put into action the first five chapters of this book before you put much effort into this section.

By the way, I was "applying" the first five chapters of this book for 6 to 7 months before I was capable of adding in an active "Body Movement" program. I like the word, "body movement." It just sounds more fun than the word, exercise.

However - there are "movements" that can be quite beneficial to you right now, even if you are bed ridden. I would like to discuss those first.

We have already discussed a bit of how the lymph system works and how beneficial it is to a healthy immune system. The lymph system depends on good circulation, yet is not equipped with a "pump" like the heart muscle to accomplish this much needed circulation. We must "move" the blood for it and we must do this against gravity.

One extremely beneficial method is a body massage. A skilled massotherapist can help to get that blood flowing and aid in ridding your system of a great deal of toxicity. Many Massotherapists will even make house calls!

Another method was first described in one of the writings of Edgar Cayce. His method for getting that blood to flow through the lymph system was using a slant board. You lie on the slant board at a perfect 45 degree angle, head down, for 20 minutes. This will circulate the blood and aid in cleansing toxicity. He furthered this "exercise" with the use of Castor Oil packs. You soak pure flannel (white with no dyes) in pure castor oil. (Castor oil must be cold pressed with no additives. You can purchase it at any health food store.) You then lay this pack on specific areas. Either areas of pain, soreness or pick a major organ, such as the spleen or liver. You then put moist heat over the pack. Lying down, again on a slant board at a 45 degree angle, you allow this to soak into the skin for 20 minutes. (CAUTION: Never use the slant board for more than 20 minutes!)

If you use the castor pack, immediately take a warm bath with Epsom salt or baking soda. The bath is extremely important as the pack breaks up a great deal of poisons in the system and brings it up through the skin (your largest elimination organ) You will literally "see" residue at the bottom of your tub by the way.

If you do not own a slant board and cannot afford one, an alternative can be found. (One nice thing about having been broke all the time, it allows for you to be creative in finding substitutions!) I used my ironing board. I put the small end on a sturdy chair and the wide end on the floor making sure the board was at a 45% angle. Then I laid on the board with a small pillow under my head. It works just fine!

Also, castor oil can stain. Cover the board with an old towel and either be naked or wear old clothes.

Another "body movement" you can do, regardless of your current health is stretching. You can stretch up, away from the floor (bed, couch, chair) working your body against gravity in simple movements. Simply lift and stretch and hold each part of your body that you can move. Do this on a regular basis: at least one time a day. As you stretch, practice some of the breathing techniques already described.

Remember, just because you can't get out to an aerobics class or do 50 pushups, doesn't mean you should just lay there. YOU MUST MOVE!

Now, let's talk about body movement for those who are not in bed. Does it have to hurt? No. Does it have to be a chore? No. Does it have to take discipline? Yes. But I promise it won't be so bad.

First thing I would like to suggest. Eliminate from your thinking any kind of goal, except time, from your choice in exercise. What do I mean by that? Do not count repetitions, do not set goals for 1 mile, 2 miles and so on. What you want is a body movement program that you will:

1. Perform for a minimum of 20 minutes

2. Prepare to increase the 20 minutes to one hour

3. Perform 4 times a week (This is a must!)

4. Create a body movement program just for you!

5. Create a body movement program that brings a smile to your face. (Make it fun!)

6. Include 3 parts to your program (this is also an absolute must!)

Part one: Warm up

Part two: Cardiorespiratory activity

Part three: Cool down

WARM UP

A warm up is required. Warming up means you are warming up both your muscles and your blood. It "mentally" prepares (if you will) your body for more rigorous activity. A warm up can include, slow dancing, yoga, stretching, walking, anything you can do to move your body in slow, non-jerking movements to bring about a warming to your muscles.

How long should a warm up take? It depends. You know you are ready for more strenuous activity when you feel yourself perspiring. So, a warm up can take 3 minutes, 5 minutes, 15 minutes, it just depends.

"If I spend time ("warming up") the proper way, I'll be exhausted and won't be able to get to the harder stuff!" Sound familiar? It was like that for me too. So, I did my warm up and my cool down and skipped the cardiorespiratory movements for quite some time. I was that out of shape! Who cares? Remember, except for the goal of movement a minimal of 20 minutes, your body movement program has no goals! If it takes weeks or even months before you can do much more, then so be it. You'll eventually get there, I promise.

CARDIORESPIRATORY MOVEMENTS

Remember, when we were talking about the need for oxygen and the need for correct breathing? This part of your body movement program addresses that in a big way. It literally brings health (life) to your lungs and your heart and in this way, delivers health (life) to your entire system. It is paramount to balancing ones body and keeping it that way!

A healthy heart has fewer resting heart beats. Healthy lungs breathe less per minute. Why is that good? It takes unnecessary stress off of these organs and allows them to work more efficiently and LONGER. You must take care of this part of your body or your body cannot take care of you!

Running is a great way for you to bring health to this system. It is free and you can run nearly anywhere (with good shoes!). However, I cannot run due to the weakness I still have in my back. I do not want to put stress on what I already know are herniated disks. You may live in a community where running outdoors is unsafe and maybe, like my neighborhood, is so populated with buses, trucks and cars the breathing in of toxic fumes is not high on your list of things to do. Okay. So, the answer is run if you can but if you can't, don't think you're off the hook. There are other ways to get that blood flowing!

Something interesting I would like to share with you about the reasoning behind focusing on this so much lies in the carbon dioxide/oxygen levels of the body. Again, we mentioned this in the section on oxygen. You may believe, as I did, that sore muscles and lack of breath during exercise meant I wasn't getting enough oxygen into my lungs. Actually, this happens because your heart has the inability to pump sufficient blood to the muscle tissues. So if you suffer these side effects, it's because your heart is not as healthy as it should be. Don't worry though, we'll get it working better in no time!

Also, some of you may be saying, "Why do I need to bother with this. I run all day long after the kids, or up and down the stairs to do laundry, or I have a job that keeps me moving, etc." The bottom line is the body will not become stronger unless it is exercised at a higher-than-normal level.

How hard do you need to work that heart muscle? The standard answer is that you should have an increase in heart rate ranging between 60 to 80 percent of the difference between resting and maximal rates. This is considered safe and a good guideline to go by. It is further determined that maintaining that heart rate for 20 to 30 min. 4 times a week will bring about noticeable health changes for you in as little as 6 weeks!

Resting Heart Rate

To find your resting heart rate, take your pulse counting the beats. (Either at your wrist or on your neck). Count the beats with a stop watch, for 30 seconds. Multiply that number by 2, you have your resting heart rate.

Maximal Heart Rate

One way to find this is by stair climbing. Steps should be 16 to 18 inches high. A partner is pretty necessary so you do not have to concentrate on keeping time alone. The partner calls out, step, step, step, to a rhythm cadence of 120 steps per minute. Keep that rhythm going for 3 minutes. Immediately take your pulse, again for 30 seconds, multiply by 2. This gives you your maximal heart rate.

Of course, if you cannot truly go for 3 minutes, then go as long as you can. What you need to determine is the limits of your heart. Please do not go beyond those limits!

Calculating your Training Heart Rate

Let's say your resting heart rate was 80. And your maximal heart rate was 180. The difference between the two is 100. Multiply that number by 70%. This leaves you with the number, 70. (100 x .70 = 70.) Add 70 to the resting rate of 80 and you get a training heart rate of 150 beats.

While you are in "aerobic" activity, try to take your pulse. Using these numbers (if your resting rate and maximal rate are the same as in this example, please be sure to determine your own!) you will know when you are at 150 beats. Ideally, you will want to continue with 150 beats for 20 to 30 minutes.

Remember, this is a goal. It may take a while, for some, like me, a long while to get there and maintain it. It doesn't matter how long. It will happen and you will forever be grateful.

Okay. So. You can't run? What else can you do? Walking at a brisk pace, swinging your arms back and forth is also excellent. It is also free. It won't harm your back if there is a back problem. So, walking could be the answer.

Bicycling, either outdoors or on a stationery bike is also excellent. Using other exercise equipment if available, such as: Norditrack (TM), Easyrider (TM), treadmills, rowing machines, small trampolines and so on, are all excellent. You need the heart to pump harder than it normally does, so anything like that will work.

I get bored easily and haven't had much money for equipment in my home. I also feel a bit uncomfortable working out in gyms with other people. Working out with one or more people, by the way, is excellent. If you can do that, please do, but for me, it just wasn't - me.

My favorite "aerobic" activity is dance. I put on some old rock-n-roll or a fast paced classical selection and (after my warm up) I just go! What kind of dance do I do? Barb's dance. I probably would never let anyone see me, except maybe my husband. In fact, I'm so sure I look so silly that I often times laugh during my dance at myself out loud. This laughter of course makes the whole thing even more silly and spurs more spouts of laughter. (I have fun with it!)

Another favorite body movement that brings breath and life to the heart is yoga. Some advanced positions, when done properly, can raise the heart rate and really give it a good work out.

I had mentioned yoga as a wonderful form for your warm up. Simple basic yoga moves are truly wonderful for that purpose. I learned basic yoga and would highly recommend a certified yoga instructor in order to learn more advanced postures, especially for the cardiorespiratory capabilities.

Some forms of martial arts are especially beneficial. My favorite is Tai Chi. This form takes great patience and teaches patience. I needed to learn patience and so it was beneficial on many levels for me. Tai Chi is much like dancing. This is a discipline, that for me, I truly needed the guidance of a patient teacher. I was lucky to find such a person and have since been in love with this form of movement. This and dancing are my absolute favorite!

Experiment. Find something you enjoy doing. Anything to pump that heart will work. Many of us have not had good experiences in the past with exercise or have haunted memories from our school gym days. Don't let that stand in your way. Trust me here, there is some form of aerobic activity available that once you try it, you'll love it. Use your imagination and make something up if you like. The main thing is that you understand why you need to do this, and just do it! (Not a sneaker advertisement)

Cool Down

After you have completed your "aerobic" conditioning or your cardiorespiratory training, you must do a cool down. During your aerobic period great amounts of blood have been pushed and pulled into your muscle tissue. Your muscles needed the extra oxygen (in the blood) in order to perform these tasks. This blood needs a few minutes to recognize that it is no longer needed in such great amounts and needs some time to redistribute itself around the body. You should spend at least 5 to 10 minutes with slow moving action to expedite this along. The best thing is to walk. Walk around the house, around the kitchen table, wherever, just walk. Keep walking until you feel your heart slowing down and getting back to its normal rate.

If you do not cool down, you will get stiffness in your muscles like you never knew before! All that warm blood pooled itself there, full of the toxicity you kicked up, and its just laying there! Cooling down eliminates this and helps the body to rid itself of the toxic residue. (It is so wonderful to use the gift of exercise as another form of cleansing. It really works wonders!)

Another thing that could happen, if you don't cool down, is you could faint. You have too much blood in one place and not enough in another and on top of that your body is heated more. So, please, cool down!

One word of caution about beginning a body movement program. You may want to consult with your doctor especially if you have been seriously ill for a long time. There may be some activities that you should avoid.

Nevertheless, body movement, on some level, on a consistent basis (20 minutes to one hour four times a week) is necessary if you are to fully regain your health and if you hope to maintain it!

CONCLUSION

I should entitle this section as a "summary" as I find no conclusions in balancing my health. It is my sincere hope that you too have come to this realization. The process of healing is always that. A process. The body is organic, and as such, is in a constant state of change. I seek harmony and balance (I hope you do too).

This new sense of harmony, this well being, continues to lead me into even more experiments with "alternative health" practices. I am concluding this book at this point for two reasons. One, the content is more than sufficient, if you apply it, to bring harmony to your well being. You will (I have no doubts) reach a place of health that you have never experienced before. I myself look and feel healthier and more vibrant than I did in my early 20's! It's such a God-send to live life full of energy and void of pain! Two, the experiments I am currently subjecting myself to, are just that, experiments. I have not applied them long enough for me to feel comfortable in personally recommending them to you.

What else could I be doing? Well, there's some really terrific healing techniques and specific herbs that interest me and I'm not sure yet if I need them and won't until I try them. When you feel as good as I do (and have my personality) you start to wonder if you could feel even better. And so I continue to search and experiment. Maybe I could discuss these experiences in another book or maybe a newsletter? Who knows?

Bach's Flower Remedies, Rebirthing, Reiki, cleansing oneself of parasites and/or heavy metals are all of current interest. Learning more about the properties of amino acids, the endocrine glands and gaining even more insight into food chemistry are also of current study for me. God willing, I will have an opportunity to share all of this with you as well.

Some people say my healthy balance is the result of my spiritual growth. Some say it is due to my learning how to be creative and exploring the wonderful world of laughter. Some say it came about because of the blue green algae, or the enzymes, or the other food supplements. Some say it all came about with an exercise program. Some say it's due to my change of thinking and how I respond to stress now.

They are all correct. But not one facet of the knowledge I received and then applied to my daily life was the answer. It was the whole program. This is a truth that I continue to relay as I speak at the Wellness Workshops I have been offering these past few years.

The people I meet now, who didn't know me when I was flat on my back, look at my life, the smile in my eyes, the bounce in my step, and say, "Barb, you're so lucky!"

Let me share with you a poster I saw recently:

> LOST
>
> Brown & Black Mixed Dog
>
> Blind in one eye
>
> Missing a leg
>
> Tip of tail bitten off
>
> Answers to the name
>
> **LUCKY**

I invite you to reread this book, at least try to find what will work for your body, experiment with it and change it to suit your needs. I invite you to end up being called, Lucky.

To your health!

Barbara Mascio

PRODUCT INFORMATION

It is not possible to list brand names or the specific suppliers of the products I used and wrote about in this book. If you would like to use the exact same products that I used please phone:

216-476-7915

contact the person who shared this book with you!

Dear Reader,

Richard and I would love to hear from you. If you would like to write; whether you have questions, comments or perhaps your own story to share, then write:

Barbara and Richard Mascio

P.O. Box 110331

Cleveland, Ohio 44111

We will respond to each letter! (Be patient with us!)

SUGGESTED READING

I have read a number of books, magazines, articles and so on. I have absorbed the material I have read from several authors and integrated their knowledge, theories, insights and advice. The knowledge I have learned from these fine authors have helped me to develop personal truths. I have been influenced by many authors, the following in particular. I highly recommend reading anything written by these men and women.

The Bible (Amplified Version)
Dr. Vicktor Frankl
Joseph Fabry
Maya Angelou
Edgar Cayce
Mary Summer Rain
Harvey and Marilyn Diamond
J.B. Phillips

Deepak Chopra, M.D.
Sun Bear
Miyamoto Musashi
Majid Ali, M.D.
Neenyah Ostrom
Dr. Bernard Jenson
Vicktoras Kulvinskas

Order Form
Complete and mail to Harmony Publishing

Yes! I would love to have a copy of "Auto Immune Illness" "Playing the Hand Life Dealt and Winning the JACKPOT!" I am enclosing check (or money order) in the amount of $10.95 plus $3.50 shipping and handling for a total of: $14.45. (Ohio residents MUST include 7% sales tax)

NAME:_____

Please Print

ADDRESS_____

Street - Apt

_____

City - State - Zip

PHONE_____

Please call Harmony Publishing at: 1-888-442-3437 to inquire about discounts for larger orders!

If you are not 100% satisfied please return the book within 30 days for a full refund.

NOTES